Words of Praise for *The TOPS Way to Weight Loss*

"This inspirational book uses motivating case studies to demonstrate the power of group support. A must read for anyone serious about weight loss."

— **George L. Blackburn M.D., Ph.D.,** associate director, division of nutrition, Harvard Medical School

"This book weaves together wise and insightful advice from Dr. Rankin with stories of success and inspiration from real people leading real lives who have really lost weight. Heartfelt tales of pain, resilience, coping, and ultimately triumph offer hope and guidance for those working hard to succeed."

— **Kelly D. Brownell, Ph.D.,** professor of psychology, epidemiology, and public health; director of the Yale Center for Eating and Weight Disorders

"Every dieter knows that the toughest battle is the one between our ears. Weight loss isn't about fat grams; it's about motivation and beliefs. In weaving together amazing success stories, Dr. Rankin delivers an empowering, compassionate message to dieters everywhere: You can do it. And you don't have to do it alone."

— **Mary E. Chollet,** editor, *Well and Healthy Woman*

DI023068

THE
WAY TO
WEIGHT
LOSS

tops

TAKE OFF POUNDS SENSIBLY

CLUB · INC. ®

ALSO BY HOWARD J. RANKIN, PH.D.

Inspired to Lose: Motivational Stories from North America's
Leading Weight Loss Support Group

7 Steps to Wellness: Control Your Weight, Control Your Life!

Power Talk: The Art of Effective Communication

10 Steps to a Great Relationship:
What Every Couple Should Know About Love

If I'm So Smart, Why Do I Eat Like This?
(with Peter M. Miller, Ph.D.)

❧ ❧ ❧

Please visit Hay House USA: **www.hayhouse.com**
Hay House Australia: **www.hayhouse.com.au**
Hay House UK: **www.hayhouse.co.uk**
Hay House South Africa: **orders@psdprom.co.za**

❧

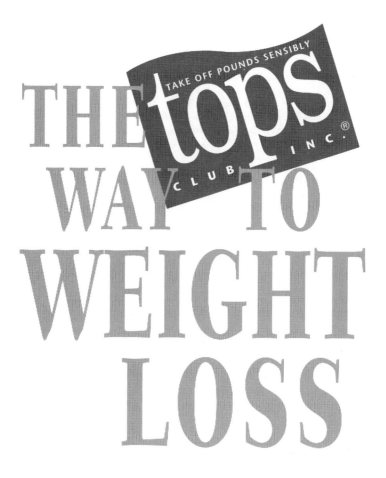

THE WAY TO WEIGHT LOSS

BEYOND CALORIES and EXERCISE

Howard J. Rankin, Ph.D.

HAY HOUSE, INC.
Carlsbad, California
London • Sydney • Johannesburg
Vancouver • Hong Kong

Copyright © 2004 by Howard J. Rankin

Published and distributed in the United States by: Hay House, Inc., P.O. Box 5100, Carlsbad, CA 92018-5100 • *Phone:* (760) 431-7695 or (800) 654-5126 • *Fax:* (760) 431-6948 or (800) 650-5115 • www.hayhouse.com • *Published and distributed in Australia* by: Hay House Australia Pty. Ltd., 18/36 Ralph St., Alexandria NSW 2015 • Phone: 612-9669-4299 • Fax: 612-9669-4144 • www.hayhouse.com.au • Published and d*istributed in the United Kingdom by:* Hay House UK, Ltd. • Unit 62, Canalot Studios • 222 Kensal Rd., London W10 5BN • *Phone:* 44-20-8962-1230 • *Fax:* 44-20-8962-1239 • www.hayhouse.co.uk • *Published and distributed in the Republic of South Africa by:* Hay House SA (Pty), Ltd., P.O. Box 990, Witkoppen 2068 • *Phone/Fax:* 2711-7012233 • orders@psdprom.co.za • *Distributed in Canada by:* Raincoast • 9050 Shaughnessy St., Vancouver, B.C. V6P 6E5 • *Phone:* (604) 323-7100 • *Fax:* (604) 323-2600

Editorial supervision: Jill Kramer   *Design:* Tricia Breidenthal

All rights reserved. No part of this book may be reproduced by any mechanical, photographic, or electronic process, or in the form of a phonographic recording; nor may it be stored in a retrieval system, transmitted, or otherwise be copied for public or private use—other than for "fair use" as brief quotations embodied in articles and reviews without prior written permission of the publisher.

The author of this book does not dispense medical advice or prescribe the use of any technique as a form of treatment for physical or medical problems without the advice of a physician, either directly or indirectly. The intent of the author is only to offer information of a general nature to help you in your quest for emotional and spiritual well-being. In the event you use any of the information in this book for yourself, which is your constitutional right, the author and the publisher assume no responsibility for your actions.

Library of Congress Cataloging-in-Publication Data

Rankin, Howard.
The TOPS way to weight loss: beyond calories and exercise / Howard J. Rankin.
  p. cm.
  ISBN 1-4019-0156-5 (hardcover) — ISBN 1-4019-0157-3 (tradepaper) 1. Weight loss—Social aspects.
2. Weight loss—Psychological aspects. I. Title.
  RM222.2.R363 2004
  613.2'5'019—dc21
2003006815

Hardcover ISBN 1-4019-0156-5
Tradepaper ISBN 1-4019-0157-3

07 06 05 04   6 5 4 3

1st printing, January 2004
3rd printing, September 2004

Printed in the United States of America

*This book is dedicated to the contributors,
each of whom was, without exception, willing
to share deep feelings and personal experiences
in the sole interest that they might help
others. This is typical of the members of the
Take Off Pounds Sensibly (TOPS) Club, Inc.
Their commitment to helping each other is inspirational.*

— Howard J. Rankin, Ph.D.

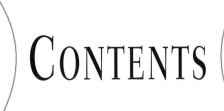

CONTENTS

✻

Part III: SKILLS

Note: The contributors' stories have been edited for space and clarity. All contributors have given permission for their stories to be printed.

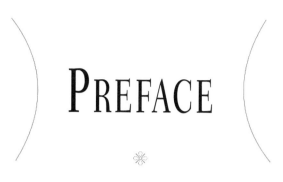

PREFACE

❀

I've been a clinical psychologist for 30 years, the first half of which was spent in my native England, where I worked in a variety of settings. Immediately after qualifying as a clinical psychologist from the Institute of Psychiatry, I landed a job at the University of London's Addiction Research Unit, where for ten years I researched the nature of addiction. In that position, I investigated a variety of important and serious questions: Can self-control be taught? Does the "addictive personality" really exist? Can psychological and physical dependence be differentiated? (I also investigated some less important and more entertaining issues, such as whether alcoholism is correlated with particular astrological signs. Answer: No, and Pisceans—those under the sign of the fish—don't drink significantly more than those from other signs.)

Working on the Addiction Research Unit, I treated alcoholics, drug addicts, gamblers, smokers, and the overweight. As a researcher, my approach was to systematically examine different treatment techniques that might be helpful. Academics tend to think in straight lines, questioning how much of a behavior can be explained by a single idea. Indeed, it's academic bliss—the researcher's Holy Grail—to find one variable that accounts for a particular behavior. For example, does sexual abuse "cause" eating disorders? Actually, about 30 percent of eating-disordered individuals have a history of sexual abuse—a high percentage, but clearly not the only variable related to, let alone responsible for, the condition.

Early on in my research endeavors, my supervisor, Dr. Ray Hodgson, and I decided that it would be a good idea to invite alcoholics to tell us their views on treatment. So, we duly interviewed a variety of clients who were currently on the register of the Institute of Psychiatry's addiction clinic. We were thinking unidimensionally, talking to the alcoholics about specific ideas and individual treatment techniques. One evening, a patient named Joe arrived to talk to us about treatment. Joe painted a dapper picture, with his pinstripe business suit and leather briefcase. Ray and I had just finished explaining our ideas about teaching self-control when Joe suddenly reached into his briefcase, pulled out a fifth of vodka, and proceeded to knock the whole bottle back without pausing for breath. When he'd finished, Joe looked at us, and with a triumphant smirk, simply said, "Treat that!"

At the time, I was perplexed and a little alarmed by Joe's behavior. Now, looking back, I see Joe's actions as a brilliant statement about the nature of addiction and the nature of life. Behavior can't be reduced to single variables and explained away by statistics. While developing techniques and identifying associated variables is valuable, it can't replace the fact that alcoholism, drug addiction, anxiety, depression, eating disorders, and weight problems aren't about statistics, they're about the soul.

It was several years after Joe's classic demonstration that I became disenchanted with the academic life. Science is painstaking, and I was getting frustrated with the slow rate of progress, the bureaucratic hassles, and the politics of an elitist organization. Academic institutions can be extremely political, with prima donna professors fighting for their turf, all trying to prove that they're smarter and more famous than their equally aggressive and self-absorbed colleagues. Often, these professors have established their reputation, fame, and fortune around one single idea that they exploit in books, media events, and world tours. These truly are people who have put all their "egos" in one basket. (As a footnote, it's valuable to remember that medical fame is based on research and innovative ideas, not clinical care. The physicians with the great bedside manner, who treat their patients as people, are typically too involved in clinical care to establish an academic reputation.)

I decided it would be more productive and interesting for me to start concentrating on people's souls rather than science's method, so I left the University of London to join St. Andrew's Hospital in Northampton, about 70 miles north of London. Now in a clinical rather than academic setting, I wasn't imposing techniques on people, but helping them heal themselves. I didn't abandon scientific reason, I put it in a different context. I used the various techniques and skills that I knew could enhance healing, but encouraged growth from within, rather than the external application of Band-Aids. I was a guide on the road to self-discovery, not a white-coated messiah.

St. Andrew's provided me with a wonderful experience. I was given freedom and the responsibility that goes with it when I was allowed to lead an Eating Disorders Unit and a Drug Dependence Unit, as well as consult with patients experiencing depression, anxiety, and relationship problems. (Northampton was also the home of Princess Diana, and when she came to open a new wing of the hospital, I had the opportunity to talk to her. She was only 21 at the time, but had tremendous charisma and vitality and captured the hearts of all who met her that day. I kept a close-up photo of the two of us on my desk for many years, and I often joked that the princess kept a copy on her desk, too.)

Four years later, I couldn't resist the lure of coming to live and work in the United States. I'd spent a year in California in 1968 as an exchange student, and as a young, sports-crazed boy, I'd taught myself about baseball by listening to the American Forces Network out of Germany, and this had grown into a passion for all things American. As I watched the turbulent and dramatic '60s unfold from afar, I became totally captivated by the idea of America, its struggles, and its history. When a doubting panel interviewing me as a candidate for the American Field Service student exchange program asked me what I really knew about baseball, I rattled off a bewildering array of current statistics that had them amused, stunned, and impressed. A few weeks later, on one of the happiest days of my life, I got the news that I was going to spend the next few months with a family in California.

When I came to America as an exchange student, I was completely captivated by the notion of those two irresistible forces: freedom and opportunity. I found them to be everything I hoped they would be—available to those who respect and value them, rewarding to those who have the self-discipline to make the most of them.

So, in 1986, I returned to America for good. I arrived in South Carolina as the clinical director of a behavioral-medicine program that focused on weight and wellness, and I combined that work with a private practice and the editorship of the scientific journal *Addictive Behaviors*. In these endeavors, not only did I learn more about the experience of the overweight and the obese, but I also developed my niche as a healer, honing my skills as therapist and guide.

This led me to research and understand more deeply the whole process of communication, which ultimately inspired me to write *Power Talk: The Art of Effective Communication*. Psychotherapy and healing are about influence, which is achieved entirely through communication. It was a shock at first to realize that I was effectively in the same business as a used-car salesman, but the reality was undeniable. As a healer, I use a set of communication skills to first understand my clients, and then employ another set to weave a personal story that's meaningful enough to lead them to self-recovery. That's the creative challenge of therapy.

In my practice at this time, I was seeing many obese and overweight people. As I talked to each individual, one thing became abundantly clear: Every one of them knew what they needed to do to deal with their often crippling and lethal weight issues. The problem wasn't one of information, it was one of application. Most of us know the right thing to do in almost every life situation—the challenge is actually putting that solution into practice. Information and education are valuable, but they're a small piece of the puzzle.

Unfortunately, the material provided on weight loss over the last two decades has almost exclusively been in the form of nutrition and exercise information. It's hardly surprising then, that during this time the population has gotten at least 25 percent more obese. Information on its own won't deflate this nation's massive obesity problem by one gram. In combination with motivation, skills, and support, however, information can make a difference—but without these factors, it's merely a seed falling on barren ground.

In 1995, as I was about to leave my position as clinical director and strike out on my own, I was introduced to the Take Off Pounds Sensibly (TOPS) organization by Ahmed Kissebah, M.D., Ph.D., the group's medical advisor and one of the world's leading obesity geneticists—not to mention a good personal friend. TOPS, a nonprofit weight-loss support group, was started in 1948 by Milwaukee housewife Esther S. Manz. Her vision, like all brilliant ones, was as clear as it was simple: In order to lose weight, people need other people. Support is essential, Mrs. Manz maintained, and so she set about developing an organization that would deliver that one crucial ingredient to the weight-loss mix.

Not only did Mrs. Manz have clarity of vision, she had clarity of purpose, too. Despite opportunities to commercialize TOPS (and no doubt make a fortune doing so), Mrs. Manz kept it a nonprofit organization with the sole purpose of providing weight-loss support. Through the 1950s, TOPS grew as fast as a waistline on a daily diet of junk food. The organization has evolved since those early days, yet it has retained the simplicity and essence of Mrs. Manz's message. Today, TOPS boasts more than 235,000 members who meet weekly in nearly 10,500 chapters.

TOPS is about people. In fact, it's called the TOPS Club because it really operates as one enormous meeting place where people share, disclose, encourage, cajole, accept, inspire, and love in order to help their fellow members not just lose weight but transform themselves. The membership is incredibly committed, loyal, and hardworking. With an enormous volunteer effort and significant financial support, they've made possible the best obesity-genetics study ever conducted. That study, conducted by Dr. Kissebah himself, shows incredible promise in uncovering the underlying genetic factors in some cases of obesity and offers hope that one day there will be medical help for a certain segment of the overweight population. For more on this work, please visit the TOPS Website: **www.tops.org.**

In a market sector that's characterized by false hope, gimmicks, hype, and outright deception, TOPS stands out like a beacon of common sense in a fog of insanity. TOPS may not be glamorous or sexy, but it's honest and forthright, and has the utmost integrity. It addresses what I believe to be the real issues in weight loss, and I've seen it work thousands of times.

Mrs. Manz died in 1996, just as I was getting involved with TOPS. I never met her, and thus was never able to talk with her about the many ways in which her ideas melded with mine. She reached the same conclusions that I have about weight loss, albeit by a completely different route: Weight loss isn't just about calories or fat grams, it's about people. It's about dreams, insecurities, fears, hopes, self-worth, and identity. Because weight issues involve these reflections of the soul, they're also about relationships. Only in our relationships are we defined, and only through new relationships can we be *re*defined. Therein lies the real power—the simple, awesome power—of Mrs. Manz's vision.

My first involvement with TOPS was to co-author a new guidebook, *The Choice Is Yours.* This aptly named book has sold 250,000 copies to its members. As I've gotten more involved, I've seen within TOPS unbelievable stories of courage and personal transformation. This prompted me to write *Inspired to Lose,* a collection of incredible accounts of TOPS members' success that tell us about commitment, responsibility, sharing, and attitude.

I'm not a weight-loss expert—I'm a people expert. I don't have all the answers to the weight-loss puzzle, and those I do have, I've obtained from others. I don't come down from on high with the weight-loss commandments, but I'm here to show you a way—the TOPS way—as told through the people who really *are* the weight-loss experts. These are the everyday folks who have experienced firsthand the pain of obesity and the frustration of being overweight, and have somehow found a way to transform themselves. This is their story; I'm merely the narrator.

"We did not change as we grew older;
we just became more clearly ourselves."

— Lynn Hall, author of *Where Have All the Tigers Gone?*

ACKNOWLEDGMENTS

❀

This book wouldn't have been possible without the wholehearted support of the Take Off Pounds Sensibly (TOPS) organization and its members—I could have included 300 stories that were inspirational and instructional, not just the 24 featured here. In a fitting testament to what TOPS is all about, all the contributors were willing to give of their time and of themselves in the hope that their stories would help and encourage others.

Others at TOPS deserve enormous credit for making this book possible. First and foremost among these is the TOPS board of directors, who gave the project their unstinting support: president LaNeida Herrick, recording secretary Nancy Best, first vice-president Barb Cady, chairman of the board Shirley Wooten, corresponding secretary Gina Brueske, treasurer Jean Terpstra, and ombudsman Jeanne Myatt. Two other board members, Imogene Welch and Nancy Marasco, read the manuscript and offered valuable suggestions. Also instrumental in the successful completion of the project was communications director Susan Trones, who provided help in finding potential contributors.

In addition to TOPS officers, various TOPS members played a significant role in the development of the book. Barbara Hartley was a willing conduit between me and hundreds of online members and helped put the word out about my requirements for stories.

A special thank you also goes to some of the contributors to *Inspired to Lose.* They made that book so much fun and so rewarding to write that I was excited about writing another book about TOPS members and their paths to success. Many of those contributors have become friends and have shared their considerable insights. So special thanks to Patsy Casteen,

Fran Drozdz, Loren Kelly, Joan Lambert, Betsy Lavin, Rhoddie Ludwig, Karen Preston, Duane Russell, Jean Stacy, and Gary Wellington.

I'd also like to thank my agent and advisor Celia Rocks, an outstanding professional, brilliant strategist, and personal friend. Without Celia and her colleague Dottie DeHart, neither *Inspired to Lose* nor this book would have seen the light of day.

I'd also like to thank several people at Hay House: Reid Tracy for his vision and belief, Danny Levin for his indefatigable energy and persistence, and Jill Kramer for terrific editorial support.

Finally, deepest gratitude, appreciation, and love to my wife, MJ; and James, Joshua, and Ellen, who lovingly supported me during the many hours I spent working on this project.

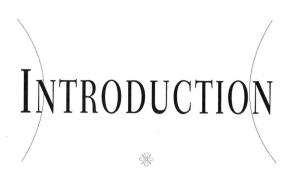

INTRODUCTION

❀

It's Not about the Food

Everyone knows what to do to lose weight: Eat less and exercise more. Most people also know *how* to eat less and exercise more—in fact, there's been a veritable explosion in dietary and exercise information over the last two decades. Yet despite this knowledge, the rate of obesity has risen dramatically and dangerously. Millions of people are unsuccessful in reducing their burgeoning waistlines, and millions of others—aware that excess weight is related to an increase in mortality, cancer, heart disease, and diabetes—continue to pile on the calories and the pounds. Research now tells us that obesity is the single highest health-risk factor, more detrimental even than smoking. (Perhaps one day, fat-laden foods will be banned public areas, as many states have done with cigarettes.) It's safe to conclude that the problem of weight management is best characterized as a failure of application rather than a lack of understanding.

There are several reasons why this information explosion hasn't led to significant positive change in dietary and exercise habits. First, the "facts" keep changing, and there seem to be cycles approximately every five years when the prevailing wisdom reverses itself. For example, complex carbohydrates were very definitely the wonder food of the '80s and '90s, but have now fallen from grace, as protein and (God forbid) saturated fat make a comeback. Salt, which was definitely out, is apparently back in favor, and so on.

Not only is this swinging of the information pendulum confusing, it's damaging, because it often provides a rationalization to do nothing or indulge in favorite foods that truly aren't healthy. Moreover, through the Internet, the technological revolution has given the world access to a vast amount of questionable dietary and exercise information, along with non-professional, unscientific, and unsupervised opinion masquerading as fact. To paraphrase a theme from the popular TV series *The X-Files,* "The truth is out there . . . but so are lies."

Second, it may not be possible to give general advice beyond the simple prescription to eat less and exercise more. Individuals vary enormously, and they have different nervous systems, genetics, histories, circumstances, and environments. So perhaps there isn't any other recommendation that applies across the board. Maybe some people do indeed need more fat, more protein, or a mountain of complex carbohydrates. (One of the unique advantages of TOPS is that from the very early stages of its development, the organization recognized both the complexity and the individual nature of nutrition and exercise requirements. While TOPS endorses sensible eating and exercising, all members are encouraged to seek professional advice from a physician or other health-care expert to determine their specific medical, nutritional, and physical needs and goals.)

Third, information doesn't change people. People are psychological beings—with the emphasis on the *psycho.* We're not logical automatons. We have emotions, habits, fears, attitudes, and perceptions—and that's just the tip of the mental iceberg. Floating beneath the surface is the massive subconscious with its huge reservoir of past experiences, memories, and primitive emotions that remain hidden from conscious view, but pull our strings like a silent, unknown puppeteer. If we were the children of Mr. Spock, first officer of the starship *Enterprise* and famed *Star Trek* voyager, mere information would instantly influence our actions. We are, however, the children of *Dr.* Spock, the famed pediatrician; we're human, flawed, and in constant conflict between primitive needs, logic, and morality. Information simply doesn't influence us as much as we think it does.

Finally, and most important, *weight loss isn't about the food.* Getting people to lose weight by providing nutrition information is like treating drug addicts by teaching them the chemical structure of narcotics. The information is very interesting, but in the absence of other very important variables—such as motivation, commitment, hope, and belief—it's powerless to change anything.

The Origins of Hope

Everyone needs motivation, commitment, hope, and belief—yet where do they come from? For some people, these critical characteristics reside close to the surface of their everyday functioning, while for others, they lay dormant in the far outer reaches of the soul. When these four essential elements are removed from the center of a person's being, depression, self-destruction, and even death are surely close at hand.

So how can these four elements be resurrected from the embers of the spiritual fire? The answer is simple: *by connecting with other people.* While working with TOPS, I've really come to understand the power and meaning of the phrase "You alone can do it, but you can't do it alone." There's no more powerful influence than a good group. After all, self-perceptions are molded in the context of the family, which is the primary and most significant group in most people's lives. Those perceptions, especially the destructive ones, are best and most easily redefined in the context of a positive circle of friends, which can become a surrogate family.

In addition to the direct and indirect effects of a group, however, there's the fact that personal motivation is also fueled by interaction with other people. Sometimes this is obvious—for example, when people declare that they want to lose weight so they can see their children or grandchildren grow up. Sometimes the influence is less obvious, such as when people say that they want to lose weight to look more attractive. At first glance, that seems to be a very individual and personal motivation—until you realize that most people want to look attractive for *someone else* (even if they don't yet know who that person is). As you read the stories in this book, you'll discover that a positive group provides many crucial ingredients for personal transformation— accountability, advice, successful role models, energy, and encouragement, to name a few.

The stories here are about everyday people. I make no apology that some of them tell of trauma, hardship, and difficulty; sometimes that's how life is. The amount of weight lost by each of the people featured in this book ranges from 25 to more than 200 pounds. About half of the stories are written by the contributors themselves, the remainder are written by me, depending on whether they felt comfortable penning their own story or preferred to tell it through me. I edited all the accounts for length and clarity, and included a byline to distinguish the writer from myself.

Weight-Loss Advice in Context

Weight-loss advice, like any advice, is given free of context. For example, the prescription to exercise more and eat less is given as a general recommendation that seems simple to follow. Life isn't context free, however. We lead enormously complex, stressful, and busy lives. Walking 30 minutes a day sounds easy, but not if you're the working mother of four children, one of whom needs constant hospitalization for a crippling and life-threatening disease (which is the remarkable circumstance of Kathy Clark, featured later in the book). Neither is it easy to walk 30 minutes a day if you have disabling arthritis, live in an unsafe neighborhood, or if the temperature outside is 110 degrees. It's my hope that by reading about how techniques can be adapted to different circumstances, you'll be able to more easily see how you can fit them to your needs.

You don't need superhuman courage or power to incorporate the techniques put forth in this book into your life. Taken individually, they're all very mundane: Walking is a natural activity, drinking water is as instinctive as breathing, and refusing French fries or driving past your favorite junk-food establishment—even throwing food away—requires no Olympian strength. Yet these actions do demand a variety of psychological characteristics: motivation, self-control, awareness, organization, planning, belief, coping, and support. Without these characteristics, calories and aerobics are irrelevant. While collectively these few simple adjustments can transform your life—lengthening it and improving its quality—to focus solely on exercise and nutrition information is to put the cart before the horse.

The Critical MASS

One of the wonderful aspects of TOPS is that it recognizes the individual variations in nutrition and exercise and doesn't set down hard-and-fast rules for its members. TOPS is a weight-loss support group, so it concerns itself more with weight-loss support than exact numbers of calories or the minutiae of exercise routines. Such information is available and discussed at many meetings, of course, but the main purpose of the organization is to help people *apply* and *implement* their particular program, rather than supply them with one. In that sense, TOPS is more about inspiration and support than junk food and biceps curls.

Of course, if you're still hung up on the informational question of what constitutes a successful weight-loss regime, the simple answer can be found in almost every story contained herein. Simply put, these behaviors are as follows:

- Reduce fat grams to less than 40 per day.
- Exercise four times a week (or more) for at least 45 minutes.
- Drink at least 64 fluid ounces of water a day.
- Eat smaller portions.

You knew this already! Which makes the above a good demonstration of the limitation of information.

Still, while nutrition and exercise prescriptions vary widely from individual to individual, psychological prescriptions don't. The key mental ingredients for successful weight loss are **m**otivation, **a**ttitudes, **s**kills, and **s**upport (MASS). Part I of this book focuses on support and motivation: The two chapters in this section provide the foundation on which the rest of the book is based, and they draw on the experiences of some TOPS members for their insight and power. Part II contains 12 personal stories that emphasize essential weight-loss *attitudes,* while Part III shifts the focus with 12 personal accounts that center on essential weight-loss *skills.* The chapters in Part II and III end with commentary by me, including five specific steps to help you develop these four critical components of weight loss (motivation, attitudes, skills, and support).

All of the people featured in this book are members of TOPS. As background, you need to know that TOPS currently has 235,000 members meeting in about 10,500 chapters, mainly in the U.S. and Canada. The meeting format is pretty much the same everywhere: Following weigh-in, members report their progress to the group. Then there's a program presented by members on a topic of relevance and a roundtable discussion of the week's progress, followed by an exchange of suggestions, advice, and encouragement on how to succeed in the following week. There are often contests, games, and competitions to provide motivation for members to stay on track. Most important, these meetings provide accountability, support, and positive role models to help members stay on the road to success.

Using this model, some groups have achieved extraordinary results—a chapter of 137 members in Valdosta, Georgia, went through the entire year of 2001 with every member recording a weight loss! The story of one of their most successful members, Karen Dixon, is included in this book.

In some of the personal accounts, references are made to a variety of TOPS events and traditions. Each state has its own annual meeting called a State Recognition Day (SRD), at which the individuals, groups, and leaders with the most successful weight loss are recognized, and kings and queens, male and female winners in different weight divisions, are crowned. (In Canada there are Province Recognition Days, or PRDs.) Some states are even divided into sections that have Area Recognition Days (ARD), but everyone comes together for the organization's annual meeting—International Recognition Days (IRD)—where outstanding members from all over the world are acknowledged.

Because *maintaining* weight loss is as important as losing it in the first place, there's a special category of members who Keep Off Pounds Sensibly (KOPS). KOPS are essential to the organization as inspirational role models. The annual meeting IRD recognizes KOPS attendees, from those who have kept it off for a year, all the way up to the longest-standing KOPS present—generally people who've maintained their weight loss for 40 years or more. In the final evening session of each IRD, all KOPS join together in a moving and inspirational candlelit ceremony, the circle of light.

The Power of Others

As a psychologist, I know that the single most dynamic influence on behavior is contact with people who are or have been in the same position. Studies on influence clearly show the enormous power other people have both at a conscious and subconscious level. Human beings are social animals, and as such, look to each other for clues as to how they should behave. As a result, successful people exert the most powerful influence among those who can identify with their problems. Learning from someone who's overcome the same problem will have a much greater impact than merely listening to an expert lecture. That's why it's so important that the lessons in this book come from real people, not manufactured composites. I'll be your guide and translator, but the inspiration clearly belongs to the contributors who have real-life experiences to share.

There are no colorful photos of mouthwatering recipes in this book, no tables of nutrition information, and no diagrams of stick figures doing push-ups. What *is* contained in these pages is the real story of weight loss—and it goes way beyond calories and exercise.

"Friendship makes prosperity more shining and lessens adversity by dividing and sharing it."

— Cicero

PART I

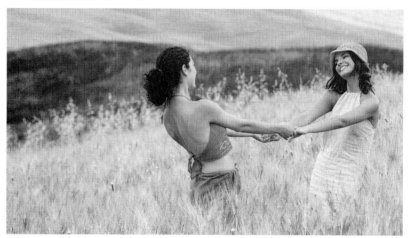

Social Support and Motivation

✼

CHAPTER 1

The Power of Group Healing

No one lives in a social vacuum. In every story featured in this book, the roles of other people in motivating and supporting the contributor's weight-loss efforts have been both necessary and vital. Although popular culture focuses on the individual, the fact is that other people are the biggest single influence on your behavior. Relationships are everything—you're defined, shaped, changed, and inspired by them. As the stories in this book reveal, there are various ways in which peers can help you lose weight, transform your self-esteem, change your lifestyle, and heal personal wounds.

In my book *Power Talk: The Art of Effective Communication,* I show how social proof—that is, the actions of those around you—influences your life in direct and subtle ways, and I highlight several social-psychology studies that clearly demonstrate the power of this phenomenon. One of the most compelling and interesting studies referred to in *Power Talk* showed that when a suicide is publicized, the suicide rate in that area increases almost tenfold for a period of time. The best and most reliable explanation for this upsurge is that when self-destructive individuals read about another person's suicide, it validates that behavior—resulting in rather gruesome copycat statistics.

But social proof need not be so dramatic. Consider what happens when you're sitting at a restaurant, pondering the menu. When you hear your companions ordering, it's natural to be influenced by their choices. If everyone at the table is making nutritious choices or ordering small portions, then it's difficult not to follow suit.

In other words, social pressure works, and it can enhance healthy goals and behavior. But this same pressure is also partly responsible for today's obesity epidemic. When you look around at the habits of other people, you see massive amounts of junk food being consumed because it's easy to obtain, can be eaten quickly, and tastes good. Perhaps you've also noticed the impact that food commercials have on your hunger, or the fact that merely seeing other people eat can send you in search of a snack. And just think about how difficult it can be to decline a favorite fat- or sugar-laden treat from Mom, Grandma, a friend, or even a stranger (as Karen Trimper relates in her story in Part III). It takes serious, conscious effort and courage to escape the strong social endorsement of poor nutritional choices.

The fact that around 61 percent of Americans are now officially overweight (tens of millions of them obese) creates even more social pressure to be fat, and there's no more compelling argument for an increasing obesity rate than this statistic. Worse, excessive weight has become a cultural norm, encouraging more obesity: If you're 50 pounds overweight—a potentially debilitating and possibly lethal condition—it's a snap for you to find someone you know who is far worse off, perhaps 100 pounds or more overweight. It then becomes easy to justify your excess on the grounds that you're not as bad off as the other person. Before long, you've accepted the extra fat. Likewise, if you see a lot of older people sagging around their bellies, having to wear excessively large clothes, and never exercising, you may assume that these behaviors and physical conditions are a function of age, and thus not changeable. That's how social proof works in an increasingly obese culture.

Social Pressure and Self-Help Groups

The only way to counter the macrocultural trend toward obesity is to set up microcultures, such as TOPS, that deliver a more hopeful message. Any organization (including the family unit) that encourages activity, exercise, sensible nutrition, and wellness is a small culture that can use the principles of social proof to change behavior for the better and establish healthy norms and expectations.

The idea of using social pressure and influence as a self-help strategy is as old as humankind. In tribal and very structured feudal societies, group influence was paramount, and there was very little room for individual variation and choice. Even now, when people enjoy more freedom than a civilized society has ever known, social influence still reigns supreme. Individual freedom allows you to choose the ways in which social pressure influences you, but it doesn't allow you to be removed from its influence— it's as inescapable as the air and as necessary as oxygen. Without this predisposition, society wouldn't have evolved.

The Evolution of Support Groups

Microcultural support groups for various social and medical ills proliferated in the 20th century as understanding of individual and group psychology developed. Alcoholics Anonymous, the archetypal support group, was founded in 1935, and TOPS was born in 1948. Both organizations flourished in the 1950s and 1960s, which, coincidentally, were the halcyon days of social psychology, including research on group processes.

The reason these groups were and are so successful is that when you're uncertain how to behave, you look to others for cues. The more a group is differentiated from its surroundings, the more cohesive it is and the more powerful the social influence of the leaders becomes. Ironically, this is also part of the explanation for extraordinary behavior in cults, where seemingly rational individuals follow a leader's edicts without question. Because social proof can be used for good or ill, it can, for example, make Jim Jones's followers commit suicide by following orders to drink poison, or can help a group of alcoholics maintain sobriety.

The extraordinary power of the group is demonstrated every day in TOPS. The stories in this book demonstrate the social processes that help thousands of people lose weight every week.

The Same Boat

Challenges often make people feel isolated. Never mind that you *know* that millions of other people are overweight, it's normal to believe that your experience of being overweight is unique. Uncertainty, anxiety, and low self-esteem compound those feelings, contributing to a sense of separation and loss of control.

Yet when someone empathizes with you, they send you a very important message—you're not alone. The knowledge that similar personal experiences are shared by other people is incredibly reassuring, and it helps relieve feelings of alienation. Empathy is more likely to occur with others in the same predicament, which is, of course, one of the main benefits of organizing a group of people who share a common problem. People facing similar challenges have more credibility and their counsel is more powerful. The identification and similarity found among group members creates an instant bond that provides a common language, making communication easier and more effective.

Anchoring

The single biggest factor that differentiates successes from failures in weight loss is resilience. Everyone has their ups and downs, but successes get up when they fall down—failures just stay down. A crucial role of support is to provide perspective when discouragement and self-doubt set in. When you're struggling, haven't exercised, and have gained weight, you need other people to restore your focus on the big picture—your successes, motivation, hopes, and dreams. One of my favorite quotes, both timeless and anonymous, speaks to this issue: *"A friend is someone who knows the song in your heart and can sing it back to you when you have forgotten the words."*

I call this process of restoring perspective *anchoring,* because it helps you do just that—anchor you to your core beliefs, hopes, and motivation.

Restoring Self-Esteem

So many factors over which you have no control influence the formation of your identity and self-esteem: parental personality and experience, birth order, sibling personality, random life events, and so on. Even the primary social group—the immediate family—is inevitably imperfect (even though children expect their parents to be perfect, and vice versa). It requires tremendous personal effort and fortunate exposure to the right relationships to escape the mold that these circumstances impose on you.

Recently, there has been a movement against parent-bashing and the habit of attributing blame to the immediate family. The thrust of this approach is to deny parental responsibility and place accountability for life squarely on the individual. While I applaud this perspective morally, I believe it's incomplete.

The truth is that parents *do* screw up their children. Parenting is such an impossible job that parents inevitably make mistakes—sometimes intentionally, sometimes quite innocently. With that in mind, I think it's wrong to assign "blame" to parents. Equally, however, I think it's wrong to deny that parents have any responsibility for the way their kids develop—obviously they do.

Ultimately, there's nothing productive to be gained in spending more than a few nanoseconds pondering who's to blame for your predicament. The issue isn't who's at fault, it's *what you're going to do about it.* Parents and other family members can create problems for you, but those problems are always yours to solve—not to solve alone, however.

Changing entrenched perceptions and ways of thinking is difficult. Individual relationships can help enormously in reshaping identity, changing attitudes, and building self-esteem, but they're generally not as dynamic as group relationships. To comprehend the power of a group relative to an individual, imagine hearing a piece of information from one person compared to hearing the same information confirmed by ten people. Which would be more convincing? It's easy to dismiss the views of one person—perhaps he or she is just trying to be nice, is biased, is in love, or is simply crazy. It's much more difficult to ignore several people.

When several people in a group, repeatedly and in their own ways, point out that you put yourself down, don't give yourself enough credit, give away your power, or sacrifice your time too easily, perhaps you should listen. When a group of people treat you with more respect than you've ever had, genuinely care about you in a way you've never previously experienced, or validate your feelings like no one has ever done before, then you're likely to reevaluate your previous experiences.

Accountability

Accountability is a crucial component of the group process for TOPS members, because it's simply impossible to monitor yourself objectively. Left to our own devices, we'll deceive ourselves. In fact, research reveals that even normal-weight individuals underestimate their caloric intake of the past 24 hours by as much as 50 percent (overweight people underestimate their intake by as much as 100 percent).

For example, keeping a journal is often touted as a critical weight-loss tactic. While I certainly agree that such an activity can reveal important information about the trends and patterns in your behavior, I believe that it's most valuable when you're held accountable by showing the information to another person. (Christi Smith's story in Part III shows how accountability can make the crucial difference between success and failure.)

TOPS exerts its influence, then, through anchoring, acceptance, accountability, empathy, validation, identification, and inspiration. These group behaviors not only help individuals reach their weight goals, they also have tremendous value in health and healing. There's much more going on in a good group meeting than weight-loss motivation.

Relationships, Energy, and Healing

There's strong scientific evidence across a variety of social species that interaction and relationships have a profound influence on health. Research with chimpanzees, for example, shows that these animals achieve optimal health when they're interacting socially and physically with other group members. In these studies, measures of relaxation as well as immune-system functioning demonstrate that social interaction is related to wellness. A variety of human studies also shows this to be the case. In general, studies with humans and other social animals suggest that isolation is related to increased disease risk and morbidity, while positive relationships are related to improved quality and length of life.

Dean Ornish, M.D., a renowned cardiologist and a leading wellness expert, believes that positive relationships are as important to physical well-being as they are to mental health. He believes that close personal relationships and what can be broadly defined as "love" not only motivate us to make better lifestyle choices, but have a direct positive impact on the immune system. In his book *Love and Survival,* he explains why loving relationships are an important part of the healing process in general and the treatment of heart disease in particular.

Support groups have been shown to be beneficial to those suffering from serious illness of all types, including cancer. Dr. David Spiegel's classic work at Stanford University in the 1980s showed that group therapy for those with metastatic breast cancer was related to a significant increase in survival rates, compared to a matched control group. Spiegel and his colleagues believe that the support group helped individuals cope with the stress of their situation, and that intense bonding, a sense of acceptance, identification, and sharing all helped the participants to live longer. Further studies by other researchers have built upon these findings and suggest that the group process actually enhances immune function, resulting in better survival rates.

Having established beyond a reasonable doubt that relationships are critical for health, some researchers are now investigating how such an effect is brought about. There are several promising avenues of research. For example, we know from research in the last 20 years that the mind and body aren't completely separate—the nervous system and the immune system are connected and influence each other. Through this mechanism, the mind influences the body. There's considerable evidence connecting stress and emotional states to increased disease risk: Individuals who've experienced high levels of stress in the three months are more likely to develop symptoms when exposed to the cold virus than those who haven't been stressed. It has been established that under chronic stress, the immune system begins to break down. Why this counterintuitive process occurs isn't fully known. One would expect the immune system to strengthen rather than weaken under stress, but that simply isn't the case.

Of course, the body can influence the mind, too. Sometimes this occurs in ways that might surprise you. Let me give you a personal example.

Medical Intuition

One morning in November 2001, I arranged to meet a colleague for breakfast. I'd arrived first and was being plied with some very strong but enjoyable coffee while I waited. At this time, I drank coffee on a regular basis, so there seemed nothing unusual about my choice of beverage. Yet while I was on my second cup, a strange thought occurred to me: *I shouldn't be drinking this coffee. I should stop immediately.* Rationally, I could think of no good reason to pay attention to this notion, although I did find it curious that it had popped into my head. My thoughts were interrupted by my colleague's arrival, and I gave them no more attention.

Later that evening, I was autographing copies of *Inspired to Lose* at my local Barnes & Noble bookstore, when, halfway through my book signing, I was struck by a terrible pain in my back and strong feelings of nausea. Even though it had been nearly 20 years since I'd last experienced it, I knew this pain well: I was having a kidney-stone attack. I got my initial relief from an emergency-room physician and two Demerol shots, and later from a urologist, who told me that, among other things, coffee can contribute significantly to these types of attacks. It was then that I recalled the curious thought I'd had to stop drinking coffee on the morning of my attack.

I can't prove that my body, aware that there was a problem with my kidneys and knowing that coffee could exacerbate it, generated the message, but it makes sense to me that this type of communication could occur. After all, the body does give us warning signs: It makes us aware that we're hungry or thirsty, and often before women are aware they're pregnant, they experience strong cravings for foods they typically don't eat—the body's way of ensuring that the nutrition necessary for healthy fetal development is acquired. So why can't the body actually generate a thought, especially when it knows danger is at hand? The problem might be that we human beings have lost—or have never developed—the intuition to really listen to our bodies. This has important implications for weight loss and other wellness activities.

The recognition that mind and body are intimately interconnected has led to some interesting developments in the area of personal relationships and health. Two researchers at the University of Arizona Human Energy Systems Laboratory, Linda G. S. Russek and Gary E. R. Schwartz, believe that the heart generates several different types of energy: electrical, magnetic, and thermal. They believe that such energy conveys information to different parts of the body. What's particularly interesting is that these two researchers believe that such energy doesn't just remain contained within the skin, it emanates out of the body. This raises the possibility that heart energy from one individual may influence the energy of another individual. As they state:

We must entertain the hypothesis that if two people are in the same room (though being in the same room is not required per se), patterns of cardiac energy travel between them, from Person A to Person B. Since both people are open dynamic systems, and since both people have functioning hearts, both people will generate cardiac energy patterns that extend into space, and these patterns may interact with one another in complex ways (even, in theory, when the people are separated by distance). [Russek and Schwartz, 1996, p. 13]

While such a hypothesis has yet to be proven, it's a reflection of the development of thinking that such ideas are even considered, much less formally researched. The fact is, we don't know the many ways in which one individual can affect another's health and well-being. We just know that it can—and does—happen.

It's a common experience for positive interaction to provide an immediate sense of well-being. This good feeling is presumably underpinned by biochemical changes, such as release of endorphins, which are related to optimal health. Feeling well mentally is correlated with being well physically, and the converse is true as well—psychological blues are related to physical sickness. Whether the influence of other people is mediated directly by physical energy (as suggested by Russek and Schwartz) or indirectly through psychological mechanisms that impact the immune system—or both—remains to be seen.

The Energizing Power of the Group

Positive social interaction that increases mood and health can come in many forms. Helping others, being accepted, laughing, sharing experiences, listening to stories, cooperating, working together on the same task, and identifying with another person are all likely to have positive psychological and physical effects. These positive effects not only reinforce further similar interaction, *they create energy.*

There's a considerable amount of literature that demonstrates quite conclusively that energy and mood are intimately related. Pioneering work by Robert Thayer, Ph.D., a professor at California State University, Long Beach, shows that when energy is high, outlook and behavior are more positive than when energy is low. This has been demonstrated by research-ing energy and mood fluctuations through the course of a day in healthy individuals. Typically, energy increases through the morning, reaching a peak around midday. This time of high energy is associated with more pro-ductivity, a more positive attitude, and an increased ability to cope with problems. When energy slumps, however, people become grumpier, more negative, and less able to cope. Interestingly, low-energy times—usually around four in the afternoon and ten in the evening—are the times most associated with bingeing.

The more energy you have, the more effective you are. If positive social interaction provides energy, it therefore also improves functioning and effectiveness. Conversely, depression is, first and foremost, a loss of energy. When people are depressed, they isolate themselves, losing the chance for an increase in energy that would come from positive social interaction. When forced into social situations, many depressives actually start to feel better. In the stories in this book, there are several examples of fairly isolated indi-viduals attending their first TOPS meeting with trepidation and anxiety, only to become energized by feeding off the energy of the group. Perhaps that's also why many TOPS members are totally committed to their group and often say that the meeting itself is the high point of their week—it gives them energy. Better to feed off the energy of the group than to feed off junk food.

I believe that for many TOPS members, the group not only provides weight-loss information and motivation, it transforms them psychologi-cally. And this psychological transformation is the first step on the path to physical transformation.

"Yes, you . . . possess powers . . . which you habitually fail to use;
and one of those powers . . . is your magic ability to praise people
and inspire them with a realization of their latent abilities . . .
Abilities wither under criticism; they blossom under encouragement."

— Dale Carnegie, author of *How to Win Friends and Influence People*

Chapter 2

The Motivational Journey

Motivation isn't an all-or-nothing concept—it ebbs and flows like the tide. Its movement is influenced not by the moon, but by life stage, self-definition, and self-esteem. But, as with the tide, timing is everything: When psychological and environmental forces align, motivation is high and weight loss is almost effortless. When those same forces aren't synchronized, however, weight loss seems impossible.

Twenty years ago, two psychologists, James Prochaska and Carlo DiClemente, proposed a five-stage model of intentional change—the Transtheoretical Model. Their model was originally designed to understand the motivation to quit smoking, but it applies to all addictions and behaviors.

The model consists of the following stages:

- **Precontemplation,** in which through ignorance or denial, there's no conscious consideration of change. A typical thought at this stage is *I don't need to lose weight.*

- **Contemplation** is the stage where there's conscious consideration of change, but no preparation or action. A typical thought in this level is *I need to lose weight, but I'm not ready to do it yet.*

- **Preparation** is when specific preparatory actions or thoughts occur. For example, a person plans to join a group or buys a low-calorie cookbook.

- **Action** is the phase in which specific actions are taken to lose weight.

- **Maintenance** describes the period in which specific steps are taken to maintain new behaviors. (This is very relevant to weight loss, because the maintenance of weight can be as big a challenge as losing the excess pounds in the first place. It should be noted that when people consider maintenance, they're almost always talking about maintaining a number on the scale, whereas they should be talking about maintaining the *behaviors* that support a specific number on the scale.)

The Prochaska-DiClemente model is helpful in identifying where in the change process an individual is at any given time. This is valuable information for those who want to motivate others, because in clinical practice—and especially in the treatment of addictions—there's been a tendency to deliver the same message over and over, regardless of the motivational stage of the listener. Indeed, the original purpose of the Prochaska-DiClemente model was to help customize communication for each motivational phase. Bombarding a person in precontemplation with action messages, for example, doesn't make sense, given that the person has yet to recognize that a problem even exists.

The model raises some interesting questions. For one thing, do people move smoothly from one stage to the next as is logically implied by the five stages? The answer is: definitely not! While some people transition with ease through the motivational levels—starting their program on day one and losing weight continually until they reach their goals—it's not the norm. Typically, the journey is chaotic. Most people, start, stop, yo-yo, relapse, lose, gain, restart, lose, and so on many times over a period of years. In fact, several of the individuals profiled in this book have gone from maintenance to contemplation in the space of time it takes to eat a fast-food meal. So while it's perfectly acceptable to *aim* to lose in a steady, geometric progression, it's also common to experience setbacks.

The speed at which people negotiate the stages of change also varies. One person might be in precontemplation for years, then get a health scare and within hours move through contemplation and preparation straight into action, while another may remain stuck for ages at one particular stage. Of course, the maintenance stage can last for decades—even a lifetime—but that's not being stuck. Being stuck is continually thinking about losing the weight (in either the contemplation or preparation phase), but never actually doing anything about it, or denying the problem (precontemplation) when serious weight-related conditions (such as diabetic symptoms) are occurring.

Why is this motivational journey often so erratic? Why is it more like white-water rafting than smooth sailing? Is it because obesity is a chronic-relapsing condition? No, it's because *life* is a chronic-relapsing condition. Almost any endeavor to change behavior that has psychological meaning shows the same pattern of success and failure. The relapse rates for behavior change across all addictive behaviors are remarkably similar: People trying to quit drugs, alcohol, smoking, gambling, and eating disorders all succeed at about the same rate. Above and beyond these clinical examples, however, consideration of how human beings face any life challenge or undertake any endeavor shows a similar pattern—the journey isn't straight and narrow, it's wide, obstacle-laden, circuitous, and has many dead ends.

If you're unfortunate enough to have had a serious illness, you'll know that recovery isn't straightforward, with increasing improvement, each day better than the last. Some days are better, some aren't, and symptoms come and go with varying levels of intensity. You might have a good week followed by a bad one, but over time, if you're lucky, you'll recover.

Oscillation through success and failure is inherent in every human endeavor. Consider the process of starting a business. Businesses that survive the start-up period continually ride the wave, cresting with successes and rolling into troughs of disappointment. Learning to ride the wave is the secret to business success as it is to life success. Likewise, riding the wave of relationships is also a challenge. Every relationship goes through periods of highs and lows, comfort and difficulty. The couples that survive are the ones who learn how to stay afloat as the wave rolls downward so that they're still together when it crests again.

Many of the contributors in this book describe themselves as "yo-yo dieters." You don't hear the terms "yo-yo smokers," or "yo-yo businesses," or "yo-yo relationships," but the fluctuating nature of these efforts make such terms applicable. It's not *weight* that yo-yos, it's *human beings* that do—in everything they do.

Life, including weight loss, is a journey—not a destination. One very important implication of this vision is that you can't expect weight loss to proceed in an orderly and predictable progression. Neither can you expect that once weight goals have been met, they'll be maintained easily and effortlessly. Your previous destination will determine the pace and direction of the next part of the journey, but the roads you choose are up to you.

Self-Definition and Self-Esteem

There are two central psychological factors in motivation—self-definition and self-esteem. *Self-definition* refers to how we see ourselves—who we think we are. *Self-esteem* refers to how much we like and respect ourselves.

It's tempting to assume that self-definition remains stable throughout life, but many aspects of it are dynamic and change regularly. Self-definition is influenced by time and by different life stages, each presenting unique challenges and requiring different coping resources. A new life stage is often approached with anxiety, and is often the setting for both personal and relationship crises. For example, having children introduces many changes for a couple. It requires new self-definitions, as the couple becomes parents, and, like many life transitions, a baby brings changes at a practical level. Not only does starting a family necessitate environmental adjustments, it heralds psychological and relationship evolution. When there's just a husband and wife, there's one dyad—that is, one two-person relationship. As soon as you add a child, there are three dyads. Add two more children and there are ten dyads, and the geometry of the family just got more complicated.

Self-definition impacts weight-loss motivation. As a college student who thought of himself as athletic, being overweight created enough inconsistency and dissonance between reality and self-definition to force me to change (see my personal account in the Afterword). However, a mother who prides herself on putting her children first has a self-definition that's not related to weight, and as a result, may not inspire weight-loss change. And if you define yourself as a senior limited by age, you probably won't be moved to exercise. Change will only occur when excess weight is inconsistent with self-definition.

To complicate matters, there are many self-definitions that actually *encourage* excess weight. In someone who sees herself as incapable or unwilling to cope with vulnerability and intimacy, excess weight is actually an asset that reinforces self-definition because it keeps people away (See Sandra Hill's story in Part II.) If a woman's self-definition is "powerless wife," and she's angry at her husband, excess weight can actually be a weapon with which to aggravate her spouse.

Self-esteem is the other psychological factor that impacts motivation. It doesn't come from appraisal of behavior per se—for example, if I'm making a mess of a household project I'm doing, I'll might reevaluate my practical skills, but I probably won't suffer a dip in my self-esteem. But low self-esteem can create feelings of worthlessness that make weight loss impossible. The inability to achieve goals only reinforces low self-esteem, thus perpetuating a vicious cycle. If I see my incompetence in fixing the sink as a trait that reflects on me as a person—as a personal failing rather than a lack of skills—my self-esteem will suffer. And not only do people with low self-esteem often feel incapable, they also feel undeserving. This makes it impossible for those with low self-esteem to achieve anything, except remaining locked in the basement of their own despair.

Avoiding the Negative

"If it ain't broke, don't fix it," is a proven physical principle, in that our bodies only give us signals to change when there's something physically wrong. Psychologically, too, we aren't programmed to modify our behavior unless there's a perceived threat. This means that motivation to change, especially to lose weight, is primarily aimed at offsetting negative circumstances. The stories in this book attest to the fact that motivation to begin a weight-loss program almost always stems from a desire to avoid unpleasant consequences that contradict self-definition.

If you have health problems, you'll try to lose weight to make those problems better unless:

- your self-esteem is so low you don't think you can or you don't deserve to lose weight; or

- being sick is part of your self-definition, for example: "I'm a helpless victim to whom bad things just happen."

The most significant motivational aid, especially when you're feeling discouraged, is other people. Not only can they remind you of goals and encourage you, they can help you set realistic short-term targets. For example, at my local TOPS group, everyone leaves each meeting with a specific focus for the upcoming week. That goal could be anything—from drinking more water to eliminating desserts to exercising for 30 minutes a day. Giving people attainable targets is important, because motivation is maintained by *doing,* not by feeling.

Staying Afloat

Once a program has been established and a certain degree of success is achieved, motivation comes from maintaining the benefits of the new behavior. Initially, these benefits are distant hopes, and as such, don't influence motivation until they became a reality.

A common mistake is to wait until you *feel* motivated. The problem with this strategy is that feelings can come and go, often in a short space of time. If you wait for the right feelings, you might never get started, or if you do, motivated action might be short lived. One answer is to work at keeping motivation in the forefront of your mind by using visualizations—imagining the best consequences of success and the worst consequences of failure—a tactic that worked for contributor Bonnie Cesana (Part III).

Another approach is to recognize that you are more likely to *act* your way into feeling than *feel* your way into acting. When motivation is low, you need to "fake it 'til you make it." Acting the part—by making healthy choices and exercising—will generate motivation.

Practicality vs. Meaning

In the rush of your busy life, you make lists, check off chores, run errands, and practice project management. In a consumer society, you're trained to think practically, not symbolically; the tangible is all that matters. Happiness is completing a "To Do" list.

In submerging yourself under a mountain of everyday details and in thinking only in practical terms, you fail to see the symbolic. For example, if you bypass the fast-food restaurant and opt for a healthy salad, you'll probably feel good about having 200 as opposed to 1,000 calories, but it's less likely that you'll see your actions as symbolically meaningful—a tribute to commitment, a celebration of focus, and a testimony to willpower.

Failure to recognize the true meaning of behavior erodes motivation. One value of a supportive group is that they can refocus attention to symbolic meaning, thus bolstering your motivation. This is especially important in weight loss, where low self-esteem prevents many people from giving themselves credit for positive attitudes and behavior.

Focusing on the positive is an essential motivational tool. It's too easy to criticize and focus on what's wrong, which is counterproductive and only reinforces a negative and damaging attitude. Focusing on one behavior at a time makes success increase and self-criticism diminish.

The Dynamics of Epiphany

Motivation is born, then, by the mismatch of behavior and self-definition. When the mismatch becomes too uncomfortable, when it threatens too many painful and dangerous consequences, change is imminent.

Sometimes, realizing this mismatch and the negative consequences that beckon isn't enough to ignite motivation. I've known clients with cirrhosis of the liver who have ignored legitimate warnings that their next drink could kill them. I've had a client with a heart transplant refuse to change his poor eating and exercise habits. Many contributors to this book tell of dire consequences of behavior that persisted for years without motivational significance. Generally, this lack of motivational response occurs in individuals for whom the negative consequences of behavior have became part of self-definition, rather than an impetus to change. For example, in

Part II, contributor Sandy Callais reflects the feelings of many when she states that at one time she "decided to give up trying [to lose weight] and just live . . . life as an overweight person."

In such a case, even if self-definition does change, efforts can be blocked by low self-esteem. The feeling that *I won't be able to do it,* or even worse, *I'm not worth it,* can kill motivation. Often, however, life gets so difficult that negative self-definition and self-esteem are overcome by sheer survival instinct.

These dynamics are important for motivators as well as motivatees. The ability to challenge negative self-definition and low self-esteem is an important weapon in the arsenal of the good group leader. Remember, *who* challenges self-sabotaging thoughts is important: People who've been in the same boat are likely to be much more influential than a spouse, because they have more credibility. That's a huge plus of a supportive group. The people in a support group, more than anyone else, can deliver the motivational message, and they can keep it going.

In Part II, you'll read stories that highlight 12 specific attitudes that are essential for weight loss and personal transformation.

🌹

"Without commitment, life is nothing but a long wait."

— Steven Forrest

PART II

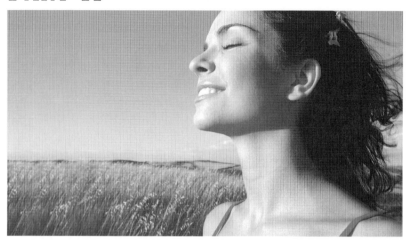

Attitudes

CHAPTER 3

✳

Resilience

If there's one variable related to success, it's resilience. Here, Anna Tansosch describes how she's been able to bounce back after losing 100 pounds on four separate occasions.

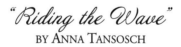

"Riding the Wave"
BY ANNA TANSOSCH

In my life I've probably lost a total of nearly 500 pounds, but I've lost weight for the last time now. I've maintained my current size for nearly two years—a first for me—and I've finally learned the secret to keeping the excess off.

When I was seven, my weight ballooned over summer vacation. I went from a child's size 7 to a 14, and by my sixth-grade graduation, I wore a matronly size 18.

To make matters worse, going from a suburban elementary school to a middle school in the city was a culture shock for which I was unprepared. I was now with adolescents who judged a person only by their appearance and had little regard for the dignity of anyone who was different.

23

One day, I was in the library when the bell rang to change classes, and something in me snapped. I can remember racing down the hall and hearing the second bell ring. I was horrified at the thought of walking into class late, being upbraided by an uncaring teacher, and standing before 25 pairs of critical, mocking eyes only too willing to make me an object of amusement. I cried and cried.

A trip to the guidance counselors' office to assess how well I was coping showed them I wasn't. They couldn't help but notice the constant flow of tears. So they set up a series of appointments for me. The thought that I had help, people I could talk to, was invaluable.

I was the oldest of eight children, and there really wasn't a place of peace and rest for me at home. There was always a crisis of some sort, and although my parents did the best they could and I love them for it, it was hard growing up in a crowd. I can't even say I got lost—I just felt non-existent. I was sensitive, overweight, poorly groomed, and I wet the bed. But with the aid of the guidance counselors and the advice of my Aunt Minnie, I slowly started to blossom.

My ninth-grade prom dress was a size 16. I tried to watch my weight by consuming very few calories, drinking lots of black coffee, and eating lots of leafy green vegetables. Very slowly, I streamlined my daily diet, until, by the time I got married, I was trying to eat only one meal a day. I never had breakfast, and I drank tons of diet soda. If a social situation forced me to eat, I'd stick to a salad or a lettuce-and-tomato sandwich.

By the time I reached my junior year in high school, I experienced another change: I turned beautiful and thin. I never had a lack of dates in my senior year, and there was no coping necessary. I was happy—hungry, but happy. I danced, dated, and starved.

I married a very handsome young man named John who didn't have a weight problem. He loved me, but was very worried about my rapidly descending size. I was 5'6" and somewhere around 100 pounds. My weight was always out of control—whether thin or obese, the same malfunctioning human who lay beneath the surface just didn't know how to face life on its own terms.

I gained about 35 pounds with my first child in 1970, then 70 pounds with my second, and 80 with my third. I weighed about 225 pounds after the birth of my fourth child, and I believe I may have reached as high as 280—at that point, getting on the scale was something I avoided at all costs.

On little dieting spurts between pregnancies, I'd lose 5, 10, maybe 15 pounds, only to regain it all again.

My weight was like an albatross around my neck. Sure, I'd periodically shed 20 pounds or so, but I'd soon gain it back. Food was the love of my life—no, it *was* my life. My eating was way out of control. I'd snack while shopping, only to get to the checkout line and realize that I'd eaten an entire bag of Cheetos.

By the time I made my most recent attempt to lose weight, I'd learned some pretty important lessons. First, I found out that you can't be led by your emotions: They're just feelings—and they make good servants, but horrible masters. Second, I learned that you can't be a perfectionist and lose weight. You're not perfect, and therefore you'll always be beating yourself up. You can't succeed at anything if you're tearing yourself down while doing it.

When I joined TOPS, I didn't think I could lose the weight, much less keep it off. The same thought occurred to others—in fact, one woman flat out asked me, "Are you going to gain it all back again?" For the first three weeks, I took my crocheting with me to meetings and barely participated. I simply wasn't sure I wanted to be there. However, the group got my full attention, and soon the TOPS meeting was the highlight of my week. I was voted MVP of the chapter two years in a row after I decided that what you get out of a group is directly related to what you put into it: If you give love, you get it back.

As I embarked on my fourth attempt to lose weight, I felt an increasing self-awareness, and I abandoned my perfectionism and became a lot more flexible. I even allowed myself to have my favorite foods in moderation, which is something I'd never done before—I would have seen it as failure. I started to reward myself for positive behavior rather than just criticize my "bad" behavior, because I learned that I can never achieve anything from a negative viewpoint.

I also made the distinction between my weight loss and my life. Previously, if I was having a bad day or struggling with my weight, I'd whine to my family or anyone else who would listen. But I'm no longer so self-absorbed, and I've learned not to take myself quite as seriously. I realized that I'm all right before I start a diet—I'm not trying to make myself worthy or become acceptable; I already am. I developed my own self-affirmation to help keep my perspective about my weight: *My weight is not my life, and it is not all that I am.* From this starting point, I feel less like I'm trying to saw down a mountain with a nail file, and more as if I'm pruning a few trees here and there to neaten up the path.

Now when I feel like eating compulsively—when I'm tempted to the point of giving in—I remember. I refocus back to the miseries that forced me to lose weight in the first place. I think back to the days after a binge— the heavy-headed feeling, the sugar-induced headaches, the racing heart, the deep depressions, the feelings of failure and unworthiness, the flatulence, and the awful feeling in my stomach. I recall the way I had to roll over to the edge of the couch and get on my knees to pull myself upright. I think about the aching feet, the guilt, and then I weigh all of these things against that tempting morsel—and it pales. Needless to say, that usually does it. But if I'm still feeling swayed, I think of my TOPS pals and how much I'd disappoint them if I gave in and started bingeing.

My faith in God gave me the support I needed to take the actions necessary to lose weight, and it gave me emotional control, stability, and security. God, TOPS, and the loving people in my life gave me a base from which I could go out and do what I needed to do to be successful. Still, the bottom line is that it's *me* who will either succeed or not.

As long as I live, I am and always will be a work in progress. While yes, I've lost weight, there's so much more that makes me a whole person. In the spring, a tree is lush and green, the foliage is so thick, and it's a sight to behold. It's hard to believe the tree could be more beautiful than it is against the picturesque backdrop of multicolored spring flowers. But in the fall the leaves are all ablaze in red, gold, and orange, and one by one they fall. When the tree is stripped bare, its true worth is evident in its root system.

The same is true with a person: Losing weight didn't solve all my problems and didn't make me rich, turn me into a beauty queen, or transform me into an Olympic athlete. But it did strip me bare as fall strips a tree. What was left was the real stuff I'm made of; I could no longer use food as a covering for all my weaknesses.

My family loves the water. We go to the beach, and all day long we get up, walk into a wave, get knocked down, and walk into the wave again. That's not too much different from my weight-loss efforts. I get slammed down, and I can either stay there, cry, and drown, or I can get up and go forward. I can assess the reason for my failure, face it squarely, and go on again, trying not to make the same mistake the next time.

A good sense of humor is essential in everything. No matter what happens in life, you've just got to be able laugh or you'll drown. Don't feel sorry for yourself; while others may sympathize for a while, in time they'll get sick of it. In the final analysis, it doesn't matter anyway—only action brings transformation.

With these insights and changes in attitude and behavior, I've lost more than 100 pounds, and I've maintained that loss for almost two years— something I've never done before. Previously, my weight would start climbing back up as soon as I'd reached my goal. That's how I know that I haven't just lost the weight this time—I've lost the self-defeating attitudes that trapped me for so many years.

I know there are no guarantees in life, and that every once in a while you get thrown some pretty big curves. I know that I may fall again, but if I do, I'll pull myself up and start over. Like riding the ocean waves, if I get knocked down, I'll be able to get up . . . I will!

* *

Rankin's Reminders: Resilience

- If I were to identify just one variable that influences success, it's resilience. In nearly 30 years of clinical practice, I've learned that the successes pick themselves up when they hit a brick wall—the failures don't. Resilience is essential for weight-loss success because success in any endeavor doesn't come without setbacks. In fact, setbacks are *necessary* for success. Obstacles teach valuable lessons, and overcoming them inspires confidence.

- Perfectionism is the antidote to success. The perfectionist can never achieve enough, and is, therefore, never satisfied. While this might drive the perfectionist to set higher and higher goals, the inability to appreciate progress eventually erodes motivation. It's fine to aim for perfection, but it's necessary to accept and appreciate *improvement.*

  These warnings against perfectionism apply to life in general, but to weight and health issues in particular. Weight loss involves 24-hour-a-day focus and many moment-to-moment decisions, so perfection is impossible.

- Human beings succeed when they're being *adaptive*. Positive thinking is fine, but adaptive thinking is better. Positive thinking implies that you need to be in the right mood to succeed, while adaptive thinking implies that you'll do what's necessary to succeed—with or without a smile. Often when bad things happen, smiling isn't an option. There are, however, always adaptive actions that can be taken to improve the situation.

Resilience: Things to Do

1. Accept that you're not perfect. Work on that attitude shift *before* trying to lose weight.

2. Be patient with yourself, and don't get frustrated if you're not achieving goals right now. Find one behavior that can be modified successfully.

3. Focus on success. Think about the progress you've already made, and make a list of what you've achieved so far.

4. Make the distinction between you as a person and your weight-loss behaviors. As Anna affirms in her story: "My weight is not my life, and it is not all that I am."

5. Identify others who can support you and restore your perspective when you're struggling.

"Always bear in mind that your own resolution to succeed is more important than any one thing."

— Abraham Lincoln

CHAPTER 4

❊

Priorities

Many people are so oriented toward helping others that they never have time for themselves. In this story of a typical caregiver, the necessity of self-care is underscored.

· ·

"Time for Me"
BY BRENDA FALK

I'm the oldest of three children, and ever since I can remember, I've been a caregiver. I was practically a second mom to my youngest brother, and all I ever wanted to do was help other people. They all came first. I always thought that caring for other people was a great virtue.

Many things in my life led to my obesity. I've been told that when I was 11 months old, I'd steal my baby sister's bottle and hide to drink it. I can recall going to the doctor for my fifth-grade physical and hearing him comment, "Looks like you've been eating out of the deep end of the trough." I have memories of shopping at Sears in the "chubbies" department and hating it. Then I lost weight in high school by total starvation, only to gain it all back. Being so fat while growing up was the hardest thing I've ever been through.

I decided to do something drastic my freshman year in high school after I reached an all-time high of 190 pounds. I lost 50 pounds that year by barely eating anything at all and dancing every day for exercise. I kept this program up throughout high school.

I met and married my high school sweetheart during this struggle. It was hard when we went out on dates, because I'd have to watch my friends feast on pizza and burgers while I ate virtually nothing. My friends did compliment me on my weight loss, though, and I finally felt like I fit in.

I had two children and gained lots of weight over the next ten years. With the birth of my son, I gained more than 50 pounds; and another 30 followed when my daughter was born two years later. At this point I weighed 250.

The weight started to affect my health: I had gallbladder trouble and was ill for more than a year before I finally had surgery. I spent nearly six months effectively confined to bed with a herniated disc. Being laid up and having my family have to wait on me was very difficult. I hated it and resolved never to be in that position again. Eventually, I had to have back surgery for the herniated disc. I reached 318 pounds, and I felt horrible and depressed. I knew that my weight was causing these problems, but I still did nothing to help myself. I remained physically inactive because I was simply too busy with other people.

Everything was difficult to do at that weight: I couldn't fit in restaurant booths or sit comfortably in movie theaters. My size made it harder to keep up with my two toddlers, and I was tired all the time. Food was killing my spirit and my body, and I was slowly becoming a prisoner in my own home. The final straw was getting on an airplane and enduring the humiliation of the seat belt not fitting me. When I realized that the belt wouldn't fit, I had a panic attack. I was so embarrassed for my husband. That event was the turning point: I made up my mind that somehow I'd never feel this humiliated again.

For years, I put myself last. My caregiving got out of control, and I'd help everyone but myself. My husband is a farmer and spends long periods out of the house, and our two kids are now teenagers who are active in sports and other activities, which requires me to transport them to numerous events. As if that doesn't keep me busy enough, I run a day-care center out of my home. I'm responsible for six children, the first of whom arrives at 7:30 in the morning. Who has time for anything else?

After recovering from my back surgery, I ran into a lady I knew who'd undergone the same operation. I told her that she looked like she'd been losing weight. She told me that she'd joined a group called TOPS, and she invited me to attend a meeting that evening. I thank God for giving me the courage to accept her invitation or I'm sure I'd still be obese. That was in April of 1999.

My life has changed so much since that night. I went home so inspired—there was hope for me. I told my husband that I wanted to be fit and fabulous at 40! Well, I was 37 years old at the time, and I knew I had a long road ahead of me, but I felt that I could lose the weight with the help of TOPS.

My newfound TOPS friends insisted that I find some time to exercise. With the experience of being bedridden, immobile, and helpless fresh in my mind, I reluctantly agreed that they were right. I started out slowly at first, getting up an hour or so earlier than usual to begin exercising.

Initially, I felt guilty that I was spending the time on me, but of course I wasn't neglecting my other responsibilities. I soon found that as I exercised more, I had much more energy. As the weight rolled off, the energy increased. Taking time for me actually made *more* time for everyone else!

The TOPS group also provided something else that was very important: I instantly had 25 new friends. After a day spent caring for six toddlers, the adult companionship was welcome. This, again, was something that I previously wouldn't have made time for.

Now I routinely get up at 5:30 A.M. to exercise. I find that it gives me energy and helps me prepare for the day. In the evenings I take time to read health books and magazines, and I don't feel guilty doing so! I've learned that when I take some time to care for me, I'm happier and have even more to share with others. I'll always be a giving person, but I've learned that I have to allow myself some personal time—otherwise I'll be exhausted, resentful, and no help to anyone else.

Now that I've lost 145 pounds, I no longer sit on the sideline watching life pass me by. I'm living my life to the fullest! I don't hate looking at my reflection in the mirror or trying on clothes. I was a size 32, and now I'm a size 14. I can slide comfortably into restaurant booths and fit into movie-theater seats, and I enjoy the simple pleasures in life, such as walking my dog, reading, and taking bubble baths.

My family encourages me and supports me every day, and my husband is so proud of me. You should have seen the smile on his face when I walked across the stage at IRD [International Recognition Days] as Illinois State Queen. He knows how hard I've worked to reach my goal weight, and he's walked many miles with me—literally and figuratively (I usually walk six miles a day). He's been with me, through thick and thin, starting with all the struggles I had in high school.

My entire family has changed their lifestyle. My teenagers eat healthfully and weight-train and run to keep in shape. Having their support helped me achieve my goals. They made it clear that it was fine by them if I took time for myself and stopped worrying about them so much.

I no longer consider myself on a "diet." I've made a lifestyle change for better health. I eat three balanced meals with lots of fruits and vegetables, and a low-fat snack. I drink lots of water, and I keep a food chart so I know exactly what goes into my mouth. Exercise is a must, so I walk or run every day, morning and evening. I ride my bike and work out with tapes and weights when the weather is bad, and in the winter I walk the halls of our local high school at 5:30 A.M.

My suggestions are:

- Be honest with yourself.

- Remember, there's no miracle pill or quick fix to losing weight. You must have the desire within to be successful. No one can do it for you.

- Take it one day at a time and set small goals for yourself. Walk or do some sort of exercise as much as you can, and don't make excuses. The rewards of exercising will show up on the scale.

- Don't skip meals, as it slows down your metabolism. Always keep food on hand that you can eat.

- You must commit to a permanent lifestyle change and let your friends and family know that you mean business. Enlist their help, and don't let them sabotage your progress.

I'm so thankful I found TOPS—it has been the key ingredient to my success. Now I'm our chapter greeter and co-leader, and I faithfully attend meetings every week. On May 7, 2001, I achieved my goal, and I was our Chapter, Area, and State Queen that same year.

Now I face the challenge of maintaining my weight loss. I know I'll keep the pounds off— I've worked too hard to let them creep back on! You must lose the weight for *yourself,* so put yourself first for once. Remember, you have to believe to achieve—I'm living proof that dreams really do come true!

* *

Rankin's Reminders: Priorities

- Not taking enough time for yourself is the mother of failure. It's impossible to achieve anything when you give yourself minimal time and attention.

- People generally underestimate the amount of time it takes to complete any task. Weight loss in particular is underestimated because it involves so many facets of life.

- Taking time for yourself isn't selfish, it's necessary. Real selfishness is a function of personality. Narcissists, for example, are so selfish that they can't even appreciate a different point of view. Taking time for yourself won't make you selfish or turn you into a narcissist. It'll make you happier and more balanced.

   When people use the word *selfish,* as in "you're being selfish," they really mean "you're not doing what I want." It's not about putting yourself first *all* of the time, just some of the time. Balance is the key. This isn't taking time from others, it's giving time to yourself which will enhance what you can do for others.

- Making time for yourself actually increases energy and productivity. As Brenda says: "I soon found that as I exercised more, I had much more energy. As the weight rolled off, the energy increased. Taking time for me actually made *more* time for everyone else!"

Priorities: Things to Do

1. Ensure that you find two hours every day to devote just to you. You can spend that time exercising, relaxing, reading, talking with friends—anything that's good for your mind, body, and spirit. This time is yours and shouldn't be taken while you're doing other things.

2. Banish any guilty thoughts. The following dream was recalled to me by a client who was a caregiver extraordinaire. Here's the dream in her words:

    > "I was busy doing tons of chores for other people. They were all demanding my time, and I was frantically rushing from one to another trying to serve everybody. There was a huge clock just above me, ticking the seconds away loudly. The more chores I completed, the more there was to be done. As I continued desperately to complete my chores, the clock stopped and a very loud buzzer rang. I dropped dead."

    You don't need a Ph.D. to work out the message in this dream: *The more you do for others, the more there is to do.* This is because you train people to expect that you'll serve them. This is especially true of children: If you clean their rooms, do their laundry and homework, make their meals, clear up their messes, and basically wait on them hand and foot, they'll expect this service to continue. Who wouldn't?

    The other message of the dream is that *life is short.* One day, that great alarm clock in the sky is going to sound its buzzer and the game will be over for you. Will you have lived your life, or will you have lived other people's lives? You decide. Know that others owe you no sympathy if you choose to give yourself away—it's your choice.

3. Whenever someone asks for a significant commitment of your time, wait 24 hours before making a decision. Too often, caregivers give their time away automatically and without thought.

4. Get into the habit of thinking through commitments to estimate how much time a project is actually going to take and where you will find that time. Too often, we underestimate the time involved in a commitment.

5. Enlist the support of others who will support your time-taking. Identify who they are and how they can help.

*"I cannot give you the formula for success, but
I can give you the formula for failure:
Try to please everyone."*

— Herbert Bayard Swope, editor and journalist

🌹 🌹 🌹

CHAPTER 5

❋

Self-Acceptance

Low self-esteem often leads to weight problems: Feelings of unworthiness can lead to emotional eating, and self-criticism can ruin any attempt to implement a weight-loss program. If you don't want to accept yourself, you won't want to accept your body. Changing low self-esteem is difficult, but, as the following story shows, it's very possible and absolutely necessary.

● ●

"Am I Worth It?"
BY PATRICIA NICHOLAS

I'm here to tell you to never give up hope. Patience, persistence, and perseverance have guided me and kept me motivated; and desire, determination, and discipline have also been driving forces that have delivered success.

In October 1989, I joined TOPS in Longwood, Florida, at a weight of 339 pounds. During my participation with this chapter, I was able to lose about 80 pounds. But then I relapsed.

In February 1995, my weight reached an all-time high of more than 350 pounds. Since our TOPS scales could only measure up to 350 pounds,

I told myself that I'd skip weigh-in and roll call to avoid embarrassment until I could get back down below that weight. Naturally, it takes far more courage to attend meetings when you've had a large weight gain rather than a loss, and I had all kinds of excuses for not going: headaches, nausea, or a busy work schedule. But mostly, I was just sick of myself and my out-of-control emotions. I was frustrated, depressed, and suffering from work-related stress. All this produced great disappointment and disgust at myself for yielding to overeating, gaining weight, and failing to reach my goals.

My desire to lose weight was primarily motivated by health reasons. Carrying so much excessive weight over the years resulted in arthritic knees that made it impossible to walk any farther than a very short distance without severe pain. My weight made it difficult to step over something as simple as a curb, and climbing stairs was utterly impossible. I needed a cane to assist me in walking, and I suffered from shortness of breath. Once, when taking my grandson to a baseball game, I was forced to stop three times between our parking space and the playing field to catch my breath. Another time, during a visit to my doctor's office, I was asked to climb up on an examining table. I was reluctant to do so, and I explained to the doctor that I was sure the table would overturn. He replied, "Nonsense, that's never happened before." But it did!

These problems were compounded by seven abdominal surgeries that left me quite ill most of the time, including two cesarean sections, a hysterectomy, a bowel resection, a cholecystectomy (gall bladder removal), and two hernia repairs. The last two were related to my weight, because I'd stumble over small things like cracks in a sidewalk, thus tearing my abdominal wall once again.

All these surgeries only diminished my already very poor self-esteem, making it much more difficult to lose weight. I was too embarrassed to go to church because when I sat in the pews, my thoughts were constantly on what people were thinking of my size. Not having decent attire that fit also contributed to my low self-esteem and my lack of inclination to attend any public functions. (Finding clothing that fit, especially panty hose, was a nightmare. When I bought clothes, I more often than not found myself purchasing from a catalog, as nothing off-the-rack usually came in my size.)

Being a health-care professional, I felt that I was a poor example to others. My excess weight made my work as a floor nurse in a large medical facility very difficult to accomplish. I'd purposely report to work early so that I could be sitting at my desk by the time the other employees arrived. That way, no one would have to see me waddling down the hall. If I worked on the nursing floor, I kept the medicine cart close to me and used it as a walker for support, as well as something to hide behind. As I distributed medications to the patients, I always had to make careful calculations as to all needed materials and supplies so that no extra trips to the supply closet would be necessary. One of my patients routinely referred to me as "fat ass." Even though she was a rather demented person, her comments really cut me to the bone and hurt my feelings.

At that time, I wore size 52 pants and a 5XL uniform top, and my hips were more than 66 inches around. I'm only 5'1", thus with such an off-balance body, I had some really terrible falls, and it would take major effort to get me back up on my feet. After one such fall, I had to slide and crawl several yards over to a parked car and slowly climb up the side of the tire in order to regain my footing.

Being rather short and weighing 350 pounds, there were a lot of places I couldn't sit, including restaurant booths, chairs with armrests, regular-size public restroom stalls, and coach-class seats on airplanes. When my husband would take me to our favorite restaurant for breakfast, we'd have to wait outside until a table would open up because I simply couldn't fit into a booth. The fear of breaking furniture or being unable to get up out of a chair were real concerns, and I avoided glassware and china departments in stores for fear of knocking something off a shelf.

On one flight from Houston to Orlando to see my grandchildren, a rude flight attendant demonstrated how to use the seat belt. She used a belt extension in her demonstration, which she then gave to me, announcing to all the passengers, "The little lady's seat belt doesn't fit." If I could have fit under the seat, I would have crawled there to hide my embarrassment.

Two and a half years ago, I didn't attend my high school reunion because of my size. My high school was a small boarding academy with a student body that was very close, and I'd developed many lasting friendships there that I'd maintained over the years. This reunion was our 40th, and my class was the honor class. I knew that almost all of my old friends would be there, yet even though I yearned to see them, I was bound and determined that they would never see me the way I was.

It was painfully obvious that my health and well-being were being seriously jeopardized because of my excess weight. Physically and emotionally, my weight was killing me. It was at this time that I made a commitment to myself: *Now is the time to change my life. I must do something about my weight.* In June of 1999, with renewed determination, I rededicated my life to the process that has proved to be successful.

One of the greatest contributing factors to my success story was my attendance at a TOPS retreat held in Winter Park, Florida. This was to become the catalyst for my life change. This retreat helped me with introspection, self-evaluation, and goal setting. I discovered just how counterproductive my negative attitude had been, and by removing myself from my home environment (even though the retreat was held only one mile from my home), I was able to detach myself from the little scenarios that had continuously propagated my defeat.

The program was very carefully structured so that it didn't permit participants to regress to old behaviors. We studied nutrition and portion control, and we had lots of laughs. Our songs and skits were the spice that made the program so enjoyable. Imogene Welch (the retreat director) and Fran Drozdz (a TOPS Ambassador) led a KOPS (Keep Off Pounds Sensibly) session, and they were so inspiring and motivating. From the moment I saw Fran, a real connection was evident. She reached out to me and touched me in ways no one had been able to do before, and her acceptance of me was total and overwhelming. I've always had a great interest in athletics, so her many awesome accomplishments in marathons brought us together. She has continued to be a great coach with lots of useful advice, helping and encouraging me both in the formidable task of maintenance and in reminding me to appreciate who I am.

At this retreat, I also made many new and lasting friends. They've given me their continued encouragement by way of e-mail, and along with the wonderful support of my local TOPS chapter, they've had a profound influence on my progress. The retreat was the starting point of my journey—a journey of weight loss and acceptance. The understanding and encouragement of all of the attendees gave me the insight and courage I needed to change a lifetime of negativity and self-criticism. Have I ever changed!

For many years, I felt like a failure. I felt inferior to everyone and unable to live up to everyone else's expectations or my own. I always tried to be a "people pleaser" in order to avoid criticism and conflict. I was always very critical of my actions, and my main thought was, *What do people think of me?* When entering an unfamiliar room, I'd feel panicky. I couldn't catch my breath, I felt faint, dizzy, and was sometimes even fearful of dying. I'd also worry about my health, but I felt helpless to overcome all the overeating. It was a very vicious cycle, and it put me at a critical health risk. I knew I couldn't continue in that manner: If changes were not made immediately, I was going to die.

I never thought I'd be able to change my thinking, but I did it. It took TOPS members and the retreat attendees to show me who I was; I could never have done it without them. They taught me to be true to my own feelings and not worry about being judged, and they encouraged me to talk honestly.

At first, I didn't know what my true feelings were. My mind automatically switched into people-pleasing mode before I had a chance to really listen to myself. Gradually, I was able to access my true feelings. I'd never have been able to do this if I didn't have a supportive group of people with whom I felt safe.

Once I was able to tap in to my feelings, I began to express them. When I did, the anxiety went away. I also discovered something very important: *When I express myself, people don't get angry, critical, or rejecting.* This discovery has been so liberating—it's been a turning point for me. Freed from the constant fear of judgment and the tremendous anxiety that goes with it, I feel much more confident and empowered.

Another person who has helped me enormously is Norma Pagan Rivera. She has stood by me and is always there for me. She took me on as her "special project" by sending cards and phoning to keep track of my progress each week. She even obtained an application for me to join the local therapy pool so I could do aquatic exercises, and we'd meet there five times a week to work out. Norma has been my main motivational lifeline. She was the Florida TOPS State Queen for 2000 from the same TOPS Chapter I attend in Apopka, Florida.

Together at State Recognition Days in April at Daytona Beach, Norma and I received our Century Club Medallions for losing 100 pounds and keeping it off for an entire year. She crowned me TOPS Florida State Queen at SRD in 2001, and we both had tears of joy at our success. We depend on each other for encouragement and support. Norma will say, "I believe in you. You can do it!" when I'm discouraged and think I can't do something, and I've responded to her gentle influence. She has been a wonderful example and has a God-given talent for reaching out to people.

Each member of my TOPS chapter has become a part of my TOPS family. They make Wednesday-morning meetings the highlight of my week. They're never judgmental when I've had a weight gain, and they're a real cheering section when I've had a loss. My dear husband, to whom I've been married for 39 years, also deserves a special survivor's award. He's had to endure my grumpiness as I struggled through some rough times getting to my goal weight.

With my new size, I'm so positive about almost all aspects of my life. I can approach strangers and start conversations, so now I'm known around my church as the "welcoming committee." The feeling of self-confidence is comforting and exhilarating. The change has been so unbelievable that sometimes I have to pinch myself and ask, "Is this really me?"

Each morning, I motivate myself with positive talk. I think, *I can do this*—and now I believe it. Sometimes it's moment-by-moment, and I'll say, "I'll do it just for today." I don't have all the answers, and I don't need them. I know that I'm human and I'll fall, but now I willingly pick myself up and forgive myself—rather than crippling myself with anxiety about how others may judge me. I've learned to look to the future; I no longer look back and ponder past mistakes.

As a result of my attitude change, I've accepted the positions of co-leader and secretary in my TOPS chapter, and I've been giving speeches and presentations at many TOPS meetings and rallies throughout Florida. Such activities would have been totally out of the question in the past. But losing weight has everything to do with attitude and determination and devotion to making a "new you." My weight loss has been a fabulous experience of sheer freedom from the many emotional and physical restrictions that excess weight brings. I'm a living example of the fact that you can't change your weight until you change your *mind.*

• •

Rankin's Reminders: Self-Acceptance

- By far, the best way to develop self-acceptance is to join a supportive group. Having a best friend who accepts you unconditionally and whom you can trust is invaluable. Positive feedback and acceptance must come from somewhere—the more places it comes from, the better.

- Low self-esteem is self-perpetuating. A negative lens makes everything look dark, and the downward spiral continues. It's important that you start focusing on what you're doing right, not what you think you're doing wrong.

- Self-esteem develops in childhood, generally in response to parental messages about self-worth. These messages are accepted automatically and become the foundation of thinking. As you mature, it's essential to reevaluate these messages and realize that they're almost always a reflection of a parent's issues rather than your own value.

- When challenging negative messages about yourself, always evaluate them using objective evidence rather than relying on assumptions or automatic thinking habits. In therapy, this takes the form of the therapist pointing out negative comments and challenging the client to find evidence that supports such a negative view. For example, if a client says he feels "worthless," then the therapist will ask for evidence that confirms that opinion. Frequently, there's very little evidence for such low self-esteem.

- Learning to accept positive behaviors and characteristics is also essential. Don't dismiss achievements, compliments, or personality traits. When considering personality characteristics, remember that almost any one of them can be an advantage or a disadvantage, depending on the context. For example, rigidity will probably lead to being both highly organized and inflexible.

- Self-esteem dictates the response of other people. Negative people get negative feedback. As Patricia describes in the above story, once she became more positive she got a much more positive reaction from others.

Self-Acceptance: Things to Do

1. Join a positive group that will accept you unconditionally. Try to develop at least one very close, safe, and honest personal relationship.

2. Avoid people who reinforce low self-esteem and negative messages.

3. Write down the different perceptions you have of yourself. With a friend, group, or therapist, work out where these ideas come from. Question whether there's any external evidence to support them.

4. On separate pieces of paper, write down your positive views, accomplishments, and traits. Put them in a container, and every day randomly pull out and read one of the pieces of paper to remind yourself of your good qualities.

5. Tell yourself daily that you're a work in progress. Repeat the mantra, "I don't need perfection to like my reflection."

"No price is too high to pay for the privilege of owning yourself."

— Friedrich Nietzsche

CHAPTER 6

❋

Self-Pity

When bad things happen, it's natural to go through a period of anger and grief. However, self-pity cannot be allowed to linger—otherwise, it will perpetuate problems.

• •

"A Sorry State"
BY MARIE WAGNER

I was never overweight until I was 33 years old. Before then, I was always active and I kept my weight at around 135. I'd been chosen Mrs. Illinois in the early '60s, and I participated in the national contest for Mrs. America. I also modeled with an agency in Chicago, even though I was married and had two adopted children.

In the late '60s, multiple sclerosis (MS) came down hard and fast. My eyesight deteriorated first, leading to several car accidents. Then my balance deserted me, resulting in embarrassing falls. The weakness and numbness got rapidly worse, and my prognosis was bleak. I felt as if I had been slapped—hard. I felt physically, emotionally, and spiritually defeated.

Between many hospitals, among them the Mayo Clinic and Forest Mental Rehabilitation, things just went from bad to worse. I reacted badly to cortisone, which was the standard treatment at that time. I also hated the numerous nerve tests that required the insertion of needles. By 1971, I couldn't stand up without falling down. I was very weak, had double vision, and before long I was confined to a wheelchair.

I couldn't stop crying—I felt that everything was wrong. Being unable to dance, be active, or go anywhere was devastating and depressing. I was in a psychic fetal position, hurt and defenseless. I'd lie in bed not wanting to talk to anyone, with no desire to take care of myself. My faith had always been strong, but now I had doubts: *Why is this happening to me? What have I done wrong?* I couldn't understand why I'd been singled out. I felt as if I didn't deserve it.

I felt very, very sorry for myself; and I ate, sat, and ate some more. Often I'd curl up with a jar of peanut butter in front of the TV. When I was well enough to be up, I painted and crafted, but mostly I just ate.

After being confined to my wheelchair, I'd take a trip once a year, either to Maine or Minneapolis, to visit friends. This physically separated me from my family, and my family from me—in other words, it was a rest for everyone! It was during one of those visits that my little size-7 friend in Minneapolis was pushing me around the carpeted plus-size coat section in Sears. It was very warm in there, and the carpeting was just too thick for this little person to push me any more that afternoon. She asked if we could just skip the shopping and go back home.

That's when it finally struck me. I knew that my excess weight was making my life more difficult.

As soon as I returned home, I found TOPS in the phone book, and I called a chapter in Palatine, Illinois. It was great! I was fired up and anxious to finally start looking my best again. The group I joined was a small one, but that was just fine. It was a real high watching the arrow on the scale go down, which it usually did every week. I'd weigh in using a 2' x 2' piece of thick plywood with a folding chair perched on it. Using a transfer board, I'd get on the folding chair from my wheelchair. The weight recorder was so helpful and patient, making this a safe thing to do. This board-chair transfer system is one I'm fortunate enough to be able to use to this day.

I finally reached a point where I accepted my condition and was determined to do whatever I could to make my life as meaningful and as pleasant as possible. I realized that I'd been contributing to my inabilities. Instead of thinking *I can't,* I realized that *I can.* Actually, if I choose to participate, I can do almost anything! The TOPS group reinforced my power and showed me how I could achieve rather than mope. I also found that when I wasn't sitting around feeling sorry for myself, everyone seemed happier and responded to me quite differently. I didn't feel isolated at all.

I'd gone to an MS support group several times, but I'd found it more depressing than motivating. That group focused on problems rather than solutions. Moreover, the stories of some of the participants painted such a poor prognosis that the group scared me. The TOPS group, on the other hand, inspired me and made me feel that I could retain control over my life.

I was unaware, however, that my local TOPS group leader really didn't like being an officer and always talked down official TOPS events. Not surprisingly, this attitude ran through most of the membership. After I was there about a year, they dissolved the chapter.

Well, during that last year I'd lost 53 pounds, so I thought, *I don't need this TOPS thing anymore.* After all, my weight was way down, and I was where I wanted to be—right? Wrong! Within a year or so, I'd put 20 pounds back on and I started to get scared. I'd lost that 53 pounds in about 11 months through a complete change in attitude, but I didn't learn any new long-term eating habits or what my particular nutritional needs were. I didn't realize it then, but I've since discovered that because we're all different, extra work is needed to determine what will work over the long run for each individual.

So I went back to TOPS again. I don't know why I chose the particular group I did, since I didn't know anyone who belonged to it. In 1978, however, I went to a meeting in Rolling Meadows, Illinois—Chapter 1846, my present chapter. I wanted to get back to my goal and be part of a working, active group. I wanted to make my excess weight a part of my past.

Soon, I was making contest prizes, helping to do research on different aspects of health and weight loss, and leading discussions at chapter meetings. I read calorie books to plan menus. Over the years, I've held all offices and have been a leader many times, and I've been Captain of Area #1 KOPS Honor Society for many years, which is a position I treasure.

But what really keeps me going is fear: I'm scared of gaining the weight back, and I'm scared of the recurrence of self-pity and depression. I've learned to manage and defeat the self-pity, but it's an indelible experience that still lurks in the depths of my soul. I have to be vigilant.

The many good friends I made at TOPS have kept me going. These people know where I'm coming from—after all, we're all in the same boat. That's what makes TOPS different from virtually every other organization.

I've maintained my weight loss for 22 years. It's a way of life now. I still check calorie counts and fat grams, but it's worth it! Never let anyone tell you that the hard work doesn't pay off. You can't compare the rewards with anything.

Feeling independent in a wheelchair may sound like an oxymoron to some, but being at a much lower weight than before TOPS lets me travel to my heart's content—and shopping is a pleasure. Having excess weight isn't an option!

If given the choice, I would have chosen a different life path. But once I accepted what I had, I found meaning in my life. I've been able to help hundreds of people lead healthier, happier lives, and I've learned patience and tolerance. A debilitating condition and a wheelchair make me focus much more on the beauty of life rather than on petty distractions, and I appreciate the overall picture and don't worry about little things.

Many people from TOPS have called to ask me where I found the strength to turn my attitude and life around. I tell them to move beyond the self-pity, anger, and sadness and confront their problems. Medical and other challenges come to us all, some looming larger than anything else. My message to you is: Hang on and keep fighting! With excess weight out of your way, you'll enjoy better health, an improved appearance, and more energy to live your life.

I made a promise when I reached my goal weight to look on the sunny side of everything and every person I meet. I told myself, *I want to share this fantastic feeling with everyone. I'm so grateful I can hardly stand it!* In fact I was—and still am—shouting it: **"Everyone, feel this feeling!"**

Rankin's Reminders: Self–Pity

- Life isn't fair. You haven't got a fair life or an unfair life—you've got the life you've got. Crying about it may make you feel better momentarily, but it isn't going to solve your problems or make life any easier.

- Pain is a part of life, as many of the stories in this book attest. Feeling sad or sorry about life's setbacks and losses is certainly understandable—it's just not very *adaptive*. I allow my clients a period of self-pity—limited to ten minutes.

- When you're in self-pity, you're sad and helpless. Neither of these states is conducive to solving problems or effectively dealing with the causes of pain. Self-pity is a jailer that keeps you trapped so that progress is impossible.

- The only way to feel better is to be proactive and attempt to solve problems. As Marie's story shows, acceptance will set you free.

Self-Pity: Things to Do

1. Recognize, validate, and manage the *anger* that comes with misfortune. Talk to others, maybe even a professional.

2. Recognize, validate, and manage the *sadness* that comes with misfortune by talking to friends and family, or writing down thoughts and feelings.

3. If absolutely necessary, allow yourself no more than ten minutes a day for feeling sorry for yourself. Chose a specific time and place, and keep your self-pity just in that environment and at that time.

4. Focus on what you can *do* about the problem, not what you can *feel* about the problem.

5. Utilize other people who can be empathetic but who encourage you to take adaptive, positive action.

> *"If you would only recognize that life is hard,*
> *things would be so much easier for you."*

— Louis D. Brandeis, U.S. Supreme Court justice

🌹 🌹 🌹

CHAPTER 7

❄

Focus

If motivation fades in and out, what can you do to maintain focus? When life gets hectic and stressful, how do you stay committed? It's not easy, but there *is* a way, as Sandy Callais describes.

· ·

"Eyes on the Prize"
BY SANDY CALLAIS

"What I wouldn't give to look like that!" How many times did I say, think, or feel this? I'd say that I'd give anything to be thin again, but I'd never actually do what it takes. So I decided to give up trying, and just live my life as an overweight person.

For years I never had any medical problems, but I figured that my weight was doing damage that couldn't be repaired. Then I started having aches and shooting pains down my arms and legs. I was worried, made an appointment with my doctor, and promised God that I'd drop the extra pounds if I were all right.

To my delight, the doctor reported that I was in excellent health and just suffering from strained muscles. Still, to my dismay, I weighed 201 pounds on his scale. I felt horrible and ashamed that I'd gotten over 200 pounds, as I'm only 4'11".

I was determined to keep my promise to God: lose weight and live a healthy lifestyle. After a week of dieting, I called up a woman I knew who was melting away her fat due to her efforts at TOPS. I joined the organization that very night, weighing 198 pounds. I remember being in awe of other members' enthusiasm and success. How could these people lose 40, 50, or 60 pounds? How could they be so dedicated?

Panic set in as the word *commitment* crept into my mind, and I realized that I'd need to make permanent lifestyle changes if I wanted to achieve what these people had. In the beginning, the idea was so overwhelming that I had to focus on getting through one day at a time. I got involved by going to meetings early, helping out, talking to people, and sharing ideas.

I'm an organized person, but I'm also a wife, full-time teacher, and mother of four, so time for myself is difficult to come by. However, after joining TOPS, I knew that it was a necessity. With the help of my husband, Mark, and my older children, Philippe and Andrea, I made time each day to walk and exercise. We agreed that Thursday was my TOPS night— my night off—and Philippe and Andrea volunteered to tend to the younger children when I was at meetings.

I realized that to be successful, I'd have to stay focused on my goals. I'm responsible for myself, my family, and 25 eager minds in my classroom. I'm a wife, mother, sister, and friend. I decided that these are jobs that I want to be around to do for a long time! I knew that to have the stamina to continue to juggle all of this, I had to take better care of myself. I absolutely needed to be the healthiest me—in body, mind, and spirit. This was (and is) my main motivation, and I was determined to stay focused on it.

Since then, I've developed the routine of starting each workday with a four-mile walk at 4:30 A.M. I go with friends, and we keep each other motivated and focused. I've been walking this way for six years now, and when I miss my routine, I just don't feel like myself. It's like forgetting to brush my teeth! I really need that early-morning time to reflect, sort out feelings, plan, and prepare. This way, I start the day knowing what my goals are and how I'm going to achieve them—it helps me feel more organized and alive.

During the day, I focus on healthy eating and the strength that nutritious foods will give my body. When tempted to eat poorly, I touch my heart and remember why I shouldn't. I like to think that I can choose to eat anything I want, and I want to choose healthy. When the foods I crave call me—and boy, do they—I try to remember what I like about being in control. I remember how good it feels to be healthy enough to walk four miles every morning and exercise for an hour each afternoon. I offer up thanks to God that I can do this stuff, and I keep in mind the less fortunate who can't.

I've come to realize that staying focused won't come without moments of feeling that I've had enough. Sometimes I think that this battle with weight isn't going well, and perhaps it isn't worth the fight. I struggle to keep that thought in check. I go through times of beating myself up about it, and that just makes it worse. Then I focus on all of the attributes that make up *me*. I'm not just the number I see when I step on the scale. Renewed in this thought, I'm content and satisfied that I'm doing the right thing and that all of the sacrifices I make are worth it.

For me, the hardest battles with weight are those fought with food. I fight to maintain the power that food sometimes robs from me. I tell myself that food just sits on the plate, and it doesn't care if I eat it or not. Its only appeal is the false connection that I've made between goodies such as cake, and feeling great. Yet when I eat these foods, I no longer feel great.

My strategy to win this battle is to constantly stay focused on exercise. I can't do without it; it has become a part of me. I remind myself that the only power food has over me is the power that I give it. When I'm strong and confident, it has no control—I have it all.

Developing and maintaining this focus helped me find immediate success. I lost consecutively for nine months with only one quarter-pound gain before reaching my goal of 128. I lost 70 pounds in all, going from a size18XL to a size 5/6.

Today, as a KOPS member, I remain active by serving as an assistant to our leader, teaching line dancing before meetings, leading exercise classes, coordinating the weekly food-chart program, fund-raising, and corresponding with members. I've also served on many committees, such as the secret pal program and incentive committee. I even developed a six-week orientation program for new members to help them understand and love TOPS as much as I do!

Some people tell me, "You look great! You're so lucky!" At first I was insulted, and I wanted to respond that luck had nothing to do with this. I get up before the sun rises every morning to walk, and I work out after school before I go home. Sometimes I squeeze in nighttime exercises. I make sacrifices every day to maintain a healthy body!

I realize, though, that I *am* very lucky. I was fortunate to walk through TOPS's doors and find a supportive and inspiring group of friends. I'm fortunate to have a family that helps and supports me as we juggle daily schedules so that I can have my time.

I'm very proud of myself and what I've accomplished. I've made a life-long commitment to health, and I work hard to stick to it. TOPS has taught me to maintain my weight, and that sensible eating and exercise must be a daily part of my life. I would never have thought this possible. It makes me especially proud when people thank me for inspiring them to live a healthy lifestyle. There are times when I can't believe this is happening to me. It feels as if someone has unzipped my outer covering and let me step out. Me—the person I've always wanted to be!

. . . .

Rankin's Reminders: Focus

- The crucial challenge of weight loss is to keep making the right choices when motivation has waned. Obviously you have to know what your motivation is in the first place: What is it that drives you to your weight-loss goals? It could be many things, and it doesn't have to be health related. In fact, health-related motivation usually doesn't work unless you're already sick. Whatever your reasons, they have to generate an emotional response—that's why embarrassment and fear can be good motivators.

- It's important to capture your motivations. Find a phrase, a visual image, a mantra—anything that illustrates your motivation and the emotion that accompanies it. You need to find something that serves as an easy and constant reminder of your reasons for losing weight.

- Don't wait for the motivational mood to strike. *You have to work at keeping motivation in the forefront of your mind.* More practice means better motivation.

Focus: Things to Do

1. Spend a few minutes each morning and evening considering your motivation and visualizing success.

2. Develop a mantra—that is, a phrase that emphasizes your goals. For example, "Fit at 50!" or "Nothing tastes as good as control feels."

3. Develop a behavior that symbolizes your motivation and goals. Sandy says, "When tempted to eat poorly, I *touch my heart* and remember why I shouldn't."

4. Each morning, mentally rehearse the challenges of the upcoming day and how they'll be managed.

5. Team up with another person to share goals and reinforce focus.

> *"One of the most dangerous forms of human error is forgetting what one is trying to achieve."*
>
> — Paul Nitze, former secretary of the U.S. Navy and foreign policy expert

CHAPTER 8

✳

Courage

Yo-yo dieter: That's how one could describe Sandra Hill's weight-loss history. Up until two years ago, that is, when Sandra finally figured out how to stop the roller coaster of weight gain and loss.

· ·

"Yo-Yo Dieter: Sandra Hill"
BY HOWARD J. RANKIN, PH.D.

During her school years, Sandra Hill didn't consider herself overweight. "I was always average. I wore sizes 12 to 14. My problem was that I was always hanging out with smaller girls who were cheerleaders and majorettes, and I suffered by comparison," says Sandra.

After high school, Sandra started to gain weight. "I started eating more fast food and generally letting myself go," Sandra admits.

Then, Sandra had a crisis in her life—she got pregnant. At age 19, she delivered her baby son, Marc.

"The boy's father asked me to marry him, but I knew it was out of some sense of obligation or friendship, because we didn't even pretend to love each other. So I refused," explains Sandra, who has a deep religious and moral ethic.

It was eight years before Sandra did get married. During those years, she gained and lost weight, but overall, the pounds crept steadily higher up the scale. Her husband was overweight and had no intention of changing his lifestyle. Moreover, he liked Sandra just the way she was—nearly 200 pounds. The couple's eating habits were unhealthy, and included lots of high-fat foods and all-you-can-eat buffets. A second son, Jeremy, was born two years into their marriage. All this time, Sandra was working as an administrative assistant at the Tennessee Valley Authority (TVA).

Fast-forward ten years—a decade that for Sandra was characterized by halfhearted attempts to lose weight, and overall weight gain. "I'd lose a few pounds, and then I'd gain back twice the amount I lost," she says.

When Sandra was promoted to a new position, she became more self-conscious about her appearance. No one at work had ever commented negatively about her appearance or weight, and despite being more than 250 pounds and only 5'3", Sandra dressed well and always took pride in her appearance. "I always did the best I could with what I had to work with," she maintains. But she still felt that she needed to lose some weight.

After many months of attending TOPS meetings, Sandra had lost approximately 60 pounds. Perhaps the weight loss itself was threatening to her husband, or maybe there was some other dynamic at play, but a few months later, she'd also lost her marriage. She then promptly regained the 60 pounds, plus 10 more.

Immediately after her divorce, Sandra relocated to another city and threw herself into her work. Life was difficult. On weekends, when her youngest son was with his dad, Sandra would feel lonely and depressed. Comfort foods were used to ease the pain of what Sandra calls "the grieving process."

Two years later, Sandra moved back to her hometown of Knoxville and started work at a different department within the TVA.

"There wasn't another person who was overweight on my floor," says Sandra, who by that time was very self-conscious about her size. Now weighing more than 250 pounds, she decided to make another attempt at weight loss. She shed about 55 pounds, but was derailed when she lost her position due to downsizing in her department.

Over the next couple years, Sandra's weight fluctuated within a range of 200 pounds to her high weight of 264 pounds. She can't identify a great motivational moment—one day, she simply looked at her reflection and didn't like what she saw.

"I looked in the mirror and didn't see me. I really had to be honest with myself," Sandra acknowledges. "It's amazing that I'd allowed myself to get that big, because I have so much pride."

Around this same time, Sandra had been encouraged to go back to school to pursue a master's degree in organizational management. There was the incentive of a good tuition-reimbursement program, and the fact that her son would soon be leaving home for college. Putting her anxiety aside about returning to school after so many years, Sandra decided to go for it. She carried this confidence over to her weight-loss efforts.

"I knew I could lose the weight. I'm smart and strong. I told myself, *You can do this*."

However, she soon became aware that something was holding her back. "As I approached my goal weight, I began the old yo-yo cycle again," she explains. "I realized that I was afraid to reach goal. I figured that if I could work out *why* I had that fear, I could finally be successful. Until now, I'd never allowed myself to succeed."

This prompted some serious soul-searching and self-analysis. Sandra recalled two events that brought her fears to light. First, some people at work had lost weight and changed in ways that Sandra didn't appreciate: "They had become so adoring of themselves, seeming to epitomize the attitude of the pop song, 'I'm Too Sexy,' and I'd witnessed them treating others unkindly in the guise of just having fun. I didn't want to be like that," remarks Sandra.

Second, Sandra had hired a contractor from her church congregation to do some remodeling on her home. She was at work during the day while the crew labored on this job. However, the contractor's wife was jealous, and had imagined that Sandra was having an affair with her husband. Sandra was already sensitive about how her relationships with men might be perceived because of her teenage pregnancy.

"I was the last to hear the rumor, and it shocked and upset me," Sandra says. "At first, I thought: *What am I doing to create this impression?* Later, I understood that I wasn't doing anything, but initially it did make me question myself."

So Sandra finally put it all together. "It became clear that I was afraid of success, not failure. I was concerned that if I lost the weight, I might lose control and become somebody I didn't want to be. Would I be able to manage my emotions? Would I fall in love too easily and for the wrong reasons? How would I deal with increased male attention? These are things you're not trained to cope with when you weigh 264 pounds.

"Eventually, I came to the conclusion that whatever size I am, I'm me. I can't control how others look at me, but I can control how *I* see me. I decided that I can manage my life," Sandra affirms. "I realized that losing weight didn't have to mean losing control of who I was. Others will look at me differently, but I'll see myself as the same."

Having mustered the courage to face this deep-seated fear, Sandra embarked on her weight-loss effort. She began by setting very specific short-term goals.

"I found that if I set goals that were just beyond my easy reach, I'd extend myself and be successful," Sandra explains. She also felt that if she allowed herself an indulgence once a week, she wouldn't feel deprived. So each Sunday after lunch, she gave herself a special treat for dessert.

As Sandra's weight was coming off, doubts and fears would recur, and occasionally she'd find herself making excuses: "If I heard myself saying, *I'll start again tomorrow,* I'd quickly correct myself with, *No, I'll start again this minute!* I also read a lot of self-help books that helped me stay focused and kept my fears from getting the better of me. My TOPS buddies were so supportive. They wouldn't allow me to get down on myself or dwell on doubts, and they were generous with their positive reinforcement and encouragement. I'm not a wealthy person financially, but I feel wealthy in many other ways, in large part due to the friendships that I've formed within TOPS."

It took Sandra well over a year to lose the 119 pounds to reach her goal.

"Everything has changed for me, and it's not just because I've lost the weight—it's because I haven't lost *me*. Getting my master's degree was great, but finally identifying my fear and coming to grips with it by losing the weight has mattered most of all," she declares.

Sandra has maintained her weight loss for more than a year now. While she realizes that there will inevitably be ups and downs, the roller-coaster ride is a thing of the past. She's currently in a caring relationship with a man she met at church. He treats her well and is very supportive of her weight-loss activities.

"It's easy to let fear cripple you. Getting the courage to take the first step is what matters. After that, the other steps just happen," Sandra advises.

• •

Rankin's Reminders: Courage

- Every choice in life has a price and a payoff. Generally, if the payoff outweighs the price, the choice is pursued. If the perceived price outweighs the payoff, we resist. There are very few choices in life that don't have a price.

- It's important to know what your resistance to losing weight might be. Most people consider their reasons for wanting to slim down, but they don't consider their reasons for *not* wanting to lose weight. As a result, any resistance remains below the surface of consciousness, subtly sabotaging efforts—as it did in Sandra's story.

  Often, we know the nature of our resistance, but don't like to admit it. If you honestly can't think of what your resistance might be, ask yourself the following questions: *When do I gain and regain weight? What circumstances make me feel out of control? What are my fears?*

- Consider whether the fears that are causing your resistance are real. Sometimes these fears are a legacy from the past and have outgrown their usefulness. For example, one client of mine was concerned that if he lost weight he'd see himself as less powerful and diminished. On analysis, these thoughts related directly to his football-playing days, where smaller meant weaker. As an older, more mature person, he realized that heavier didn't mean stronger, and he was able to release this source of resistance.

  There are times when resistance reflects a legitimate anxiety. For example, many women have the same fear that Sandra expressed in her story—concern about how they might respond to increased male attention. It's important to address such anxieties. Working out a strategy for resolving this issue—such as talking with others or role-playing—is better than sabotaging your health.

- Remember that anxiety is anticipatory, and, as Sandra discovered, is often largely unfounded. Many people worry about things that are never going to happen, or underestimate their ability to cope with hypothetical scenarios. But in most cases, facing a challenge head-on is less stressful than remaining a prisoner of worry.

Courage: Things to Do

1. Write down the pros and cons for losing weight. Identify all the reasons you might have for not wanting to lose weight, and prioritize this list in terms of which items make you most fearful.

2. Ask yourself what circumstances have caused you to gain and regain weight in the past. Writing this down may help you detect patterns in your behavior.

3. Discuss fears and reasons for resistance with appropriate friends. If you need more help, consult a professional.

4. Assess whether your fears are justified. If they are, devise strategies for dealing with them.

5. Keep your focus on the present. Remember, most anxiety is anticipatory.

"Fear is a question: What are you afraid of, and why?
Just as the seed of health is in illness, because illness
contains information, your fears are a treasure
house of self-knowledge if you explore them."

— Marilyn Ferguson, author

CHAPTER 9

❋

Responsibility

When life becomes overwhelmingly stressful, it's tempting to abandon self-care and devote all your energy and time to others. Kathy Clark's story is a reminder that such denial is a dangerous and misguided tactic. In it, she gives us one simple phrase that's an essential mantra for weight loss . . . and for life.

• •

"Part of the Problem"
BY KATHY CLARK

I've experienced the highs and lows of life. Like my weight, my life circumstances have swung between extremes. Much of the wild oscillation in my weight and life occurred about ten years ago, but for the last four years, things have been under control. This means, for starters, that I've maintained a 185-pound weight loss.

My life could never have been described as "conventional": I discovered that I was pregnant on the day I graduated from parochial school, I was married soon after, and I went on to have five children in all. Twenty years later, my marriage was deteriorating rapidly, I weighed nearly 300

63

pounds, I had no confidence, and I harbored a tremendous fear of being alone. I felt that I had to do something. I was screwing up my life.

One evening while lying in bed reading, I felt some indigestion—like heartburn. I asked one of my kids to get me a soda. The same thing happened the next night, and then the next. When I casually mentioned this to a nurse friend, her response was as sudden as it was dramatic: "You're not having indigestion, that's a heart attack!" she exclaimed, and she made arrangements to get me into the intensive-care unit immediately.

Luckily I had no pain, and all the initial tests were normal. I was about to be released when the doctor ran a few more tests, just to be sure. The results showed that I had three blocked arteries and needed immediate angioplasty. I was just 39 years old.

A couple years later, my marriage finally fell apart, requiring my five children and me to leave a large, comfortable house and nice lifestyle and move into a small place infested with roaches and even bats. At the same time, my father, with whom I was very close, was diagnosed with cancer and given a poor prognosis. His death six months later was devastating to me.

Dad was a World War II veteran who'd been stationed in Europe and fought in the Battle of the Bulge. After that, he worked 30-plus years at Prudential Insurance Company, where he oversaw more than a thousand people. I doubt if you could find a handful of employees that thought that he was unfair to them. He was loved by hundreds of people, and despite the fact that his funeral took place on the coldest day recorded in the county in a decade, there was standing room only.

My father always put his family first, and I felt like I was number one in his life. He was my hero, and when he died, he left a void in my life that will never be filled. He wanted me to be thin very badly, because he, too, had a weight problem for a good part of his life, and he'd also experienced heart problems at a young age. Yet he was able to lose 50 pounds and maintain that loss for 20 years through diet and exercise.

At the time of Dad's death, my weight had ballooned to 340 pounds, and I didn't have a suitable dress to wear to the funeral. I had to rush to the local "stout" shop, where it wasn't a case of choosing a dress as much as taking what was available. The only dress in my size was purple. So I went to my dad's funeral looking like Barney.

My father had so many sayings—I don't know where in the world he got them. But the one that probably had the most impact on me is: *You are your only problem, and you are your only solution.* When I was younger, I'd hear him say that, and I could never figure out how you could be a problem to yourself. I figured self-preservation would always be on your side. As I got older, I realized that my definition of self-preservation wasn't always healthy.

Divorce, death, and downward social mobility weren't the only traumas in my life. My youngest son, Daniel, had been diagnosed with cystic fibrosis at the age of 16, just about the time my father was diagnosed with lung cancer. For three of his four years of high school, Daniel was hospitalized, receiving treatment for complications of the disease, which in his case included epilepsy and pancreatitis. Of all my children, Daniel was the one who was most critical of my weight, often complaining that he couldn't hug me properly because his arms wouldn't fit all the way around my waist.

The reason that I mention all of this is because Daniel's illness was a constant, daily battle. When he was 14 years old, Daniel had his appendix removed, but he didn't get better. Two weeks later, he had the same pain that we'd associated with his appendix. He was readmitted to the hospital and diagnosed with pancreatitis. We saw specialist after specialist—some of the best doctors in Indianapolis—and he was in the hospital for weeks and months at a time, yet no one could figure out what was going on. It was truly a seesaw—emotionally, physically, and mentally. Finally, 18 months later, a doctor diagnosed him with cystic fibrosis.

I was trying to balance working full time, taking Daniel to all of the doctors that he needed to see, and caring for my terminally ill father. I remember thinking, *Just put one foot in front of the other, and never fall down.*

In all of the years that Daniel spent in the hospital, I never missed a day of going to see him. My reward for getting through all of those days was eating; that's how I got my comfort. I realized that I had no control over Daniel's illness, my fathers' illness and death, my ex-husband's drinking, or my failed marriage. The only thing that I had control over was myself and my weight, and I wasn't doing a very good job. I wanted to be thin, but because I had no control over the one thing that I *could* change, I had no one to blame but me. *I* was preventing myself from having what I wanted. Although I felt totally weak and powerless in just about every aspect of my life, I knew that if I was able to take charge of my weight, it would give me the confidence to handle other problems.

All of these thoughts had been swirling in my head like a tornado for several days before I had my epiphany. Leaving the hospital after a traumatic visit with Daniel, I noticed a reflection in the window as I walked toward the parking lot. My first reaction was, *Oh, there's someone fatter than me.* Then I realized that it *was* me, and I was disgusted with myself. I knew that I had candy bars in my purse, so I immediately threw them in the nearest trash can. From that day on, I was going to lose the weight.

But it wasn't just seeing my reflection in the window that caused the reaction. Prior to leaving the hospital that day, two things had happened that sensitized me to my weight and what it meant in my life. First, I'd been talking with two of Daniel's doctors. One of them had sympathetically touched my arm. It was a supportive gesture, and although I didn't interpret it romantically, it reminded me that I'd been missing a man's touch. If I was ever going to experience that again, I'd need to lose the weight. Second, no sooner had I thought this when a very slim woman passed by. Both doctors turned their heads to look at her, leaving me feeling rejected and angry. It was with these feelings fresh in my mind that I caught my reflection in the mirror.

Now motivated to take action, I joined the local TOPS chapter along with my mother. I imagined that I weighed about 270, but was shocked to find myself well over 300. Anyway, in the nearly five years since that first meeting, I've only missed going three times.

At the time that I joined TOPS, my son Michael's wedding was just a little more than a year away. I wanted to be under 200, which would mean losing 140 pounds in 13 months. When the day came, I weighed 201, not 199 as I had hoped. But I *had* lost 139 pounds.

I was able to shed half my weight—a loss of 170 pounds—before I reached a plateau. At that point, I really increased my exercise, mainly by walking on my treadmill. One tactic that has helped me drop nearly 200 pounds and keep it off is to stay on just the right side of the dedicated/obsessed boundary. I make the commitment to do something wholeheartedly and don't give myself the chance to opt out. There are no decisions involved; I just do it.

"Doing it" currently means getting up at 4:30 A.M. and walking for 45 minutes on the treadmill—with nine-pound weights in each hand, on an 11-percent incline. Remember, this is from a woman who previously had been very inactive. My commitment to this exercise regime enabled me to lose the last 15 pounds for an overall loss of 185 pounds, which I've maintained for the past four years.

I lost my weight by allowing myself to have some of the foods I like in moderation, but being totally committed to not giving myself options that could disrupt my program. For example, I keep my diet within a range of 1,200 to 1,500 calories a day, but permit myself some treats in moderation within that range, provided I'm able to meet other health goals. If I feel that the treats are getting out of hand, I throw them away. I feel as if the fat side of me is a hibernating bear, and I can't afford to wake her up.

Ice cream used to be a major problem for me. On weekends, I could eat as much as two pints per day. I was so embarrassed about this that I'd go to three separate stores to buy my supply, rather than get it all at one place. I now occasionally allow myself some ice cream or frozen yogurt, eat a moderate amount, and then toss the remainder. On one occasion, I ordered a favorite dessert, tiramisu. When I'd eaten the planned amount, I poured ketchup over the rest to eliminate the possibility of overeating.

I also set rules for myself and control my environment, which means that when one of my kids brings home a box of Oreo cookies, these are kept in his or her room or thrown away. My first response to temptation is to say no, and that empowers me.

Now that I've lost the weight, I feel good, and my health has improved dramatically. When I was obese, I wasn't interested in clothes. Now I enjoy being able to buy anything and look wonderful, rather than fat. My blood pressure, which was previously 170/140, is now a healthy 120/75. But when I'm asked about the biggest difference between weighing 340 and 155, I always reply assertively and decisively, "Confidence!"

I used to be very self-deprecating. I always had to get the first negative word in about myself before others did. That way, I had some control over the hurt. Then I wanted to hide—now I want to be seen. I feel reborn.

There's no good news regarding my son's terminal illness. I've realized, however, that I have a voice. I know that health-care professionals are very busy people, and I know that Daniel and I are not the only patients they have. However, the way I interact with these people now, compared to before I lost the weight, is the difference between night and day. I never want to make unrealistic demands, but I do make sure that our concerns and suggestions are heard, with a voice that's loud and clear.

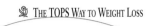

My son Daniel can give me a real hug now, and I know that my father is in heaven and he sees that I've reached my goal. And I'm sure he's happy that he gave me those magic words: *You are your only problem, and you are your only solution.*

. . . .

Rankin's Reminders: Responsibility

- Life's responsibilities can be overwhelming. As adults we acquire a lot of responsibility, and it's normal to want to revert to that blissful childhood state where responsibilities were limited or nonexistent. There are times we wish we could wave a magic wand and our obligations would simply disappear. It's a nice fantasy, but a fantasy nonetheless: No matter how much you may want to wish your responsibilities away, they're here to stay.

- You, and you alone, are responsible for your mind, body, health, and weight. You have to eliminate excuses as well as junk food. If you fail, it will be your fault. If you succeed, you can take the credit. The buck stops with you.

- If you're overwhelmed by a problem and you have an extensive history of failure, it's tempting to conclude that the only way change is going to occur is through the efforts of other people. However, as desperate as you may get, you have to remember that the cavalry isn't coming. Other people can be helpful and supportive, but no one is going to rescue you, make it easy, or save you from yourself. The sooner you accept this, the sooner you can embark on a program that will succeed.

- You can't control other people's behavior, yet so many of us spend time trying to control others while neglecting ourselves. Folks, this is the wrong way to go about things.

- Often, we get more involved in other people's lives and struggles because they're a useful distraction from addressing our own problems. But neglecting your issues won't make them go away.

Responsibility: Things to Do

1. Ask for assistance. Don't ask people to do it for you, ask them to help you do it.

2. Whenever you feel an excuse coming on, remind yourself: *I'm my only problem, and I'm my only solution.* Repeat this mantra every day.

3. It's possible to be unaware of how dependent you've become. You may not realize that you're really expecting other people not just to help you, but to do it for you. Make a list of the important people in your life and what you expect of them. Is it too much?

4. Observe other people and determine whether they're taking responsibility for the issues in their lives, and then examine your own life for the same patterns. Sometimes it's easier to recognize the habitual behaviors in other people's lives than in your own.

5. Make a list of your responsibilities. Appreciate your successes, and devise ways of improving in areas that need work.

"To shun one's cross is to make it heavier."

— Henri Frédéric Amiel, philosopher

CHAPTER 10

✳

Self-Defeat

When crisis strikes, it's natural for emotion to take over. However, it's crucial to prevent your feelings from dictating your behavior, thus making a bad situation worse.

. . . .

"A Shot in the Foot: Karen Dixon"
BY HOWARD J. RANKIN, PH.D.

Karen Dixon knows all about handicaps. The first part of her life was normal—she graduated from high school, married, and had a baby boy she named Justin. Another son, Brent, soon followed. Karen never had a weight problem.

Life changed forever for Karen when she noticed that Brent was slow in reaching his developmental milestones. He didn't walk or crawl, and he had difficulty just holding his head up. When Brent was 13 months old, he went to a specialist who took a muscle biopsy. There followed a long two-week wait for the results.

"I was at home alone when the news came. The doctor's office called with the results of the biopsy, and they told me that my son had muscular dystrophy," says Karen. Since she understood that muscular dystrophy is a progressive illness, Karen knew that her baby boy, who'd never even crawled, would spend most of his life in a wheelchair. Lacking any muscle control, he'd need constant care.

Today, Karen declares that "there's nothing we wouldn't do for Brent. We've really become a nursing home 24/7, and I've been up every night for 14 years to tend to him. I can't sleep anyway." Brent has been in a wheelchair since he was three. His mother, father, and older brother care for him constantly. He needs help with every task—getting dressed, getting into the wheelchair, rolling over in bed, and going to the bathroom.

The grief of the diagnosis and the sheer effort required to care for Brent sent Karen into a depressive tailspin. "I started eating a lot, mostly high-calorie comfort food, and I cooked a lot of fried food and cakes. I wanted to treat my family and myself; I felt that we needed that. We were all devastated and exhausted," Karen explains.

When you have a handicapped child, every experience is magnified. The lows are very low, but the highs are also very high. Most of the time, the continual demands, lack of sleep, grief, and worry led Karen to the scrapheap. But there were wonderful events that took her to the heavens, like the time the Make-A-Wish Foundation (a program designed to grant wishes to children with life-threatening medical conditions) provided a trip to Disney World in Orlando, Florida.

As a young child, Brent had been a huge fan of "Ickey Ouse." So when he was four, the Foundation gave Brent and his family an all-expenses-paid trip to Orlando. It had the desired effect: "We were treated like kings," says Karen. "It made Brent's life. He still recalls it today, ten years later."

Such moments were jewels in a crown that was made mostly of thorns. With a relentless pattern of providing total care without any relief and a diet designed to comfort, Karen gained 100 pounds in about ten years.

"I got to be 39, and I took a really good look at myself," Karen remembers. "There had to be more to life than this. I felt like I was dying inside, and I knew I had to start looking out for my health."

Karen had read about TOPS in a newspaper article on the success of local leader, Patsy Casteen. Patsy, who herself had an incredible story that was featured in my book *Inspired to Lose,* is dynamic and inspirational. So Karen checked out the local chapter, even though it wasn't her intention to join immediately. She didn't know anybody there, and she was, by her own admission, "very reserved." She'd spent so much time caring for Brent that adult company was a rare luxury.

Supported by her husband and boys to make Thursday night her night, Karen found within TOPS the support, companionship, and social outlet that she so desperately needed. "Patsy was very sweet and welcoming, as was everyone else," says Karen. "I felt as if God had put these special people there for me."

Motivated and supported, Karen started her weight-loss efforts in a determined fashion: She didn't just drink eight glasses of water a day, she drank a gallon of it. Although she'd never previously been an exerciser, Karen walked three to four miles a day, six days a week. She developed low-fat recipes and always checked labels for nutrition information. She threw herself into her program—in fact, she had only 3 gaining weeks in 42. Ultimately, Karen lost 100 pounds in a little more than ten months, going from a size 26 to a size 8.

Karen changed the family diet, too. Since realizing that fried food is toxic for her, she hardly ever fries anything. The family has accepted these changes, although Brent sometimes reminds her, "I'm not on a diet like you!" The Dixons are a much healthier family now.

The weight loss has made a major difference in Karen's life. Her self-esteem has risen, and she's no longer depressed. "I'm happy with myself," she says. She also has more energy, which gives her physical and emotional strength. "It's so much easier for me to care for Brent now. One thing I really like is that I can get up on the bed next to him and watch TV with him. Moving him and carrying him is so much easier," Karen says, "and he can hug me now."

Brent's condition was an invitation to Karen and her family to take the best possible care of themselves so that they could give the best possible care to him, but ironically, Karen's initial response to this difficult situation was to do the opposite. Sometimes the very aspects of life that should be the invitation to pursue health turn out to be the very reasons we don't.

"I wish I'd lost the weight sooner—or never gained it in the first place," she says. "Now, my increased ability to care for Brent is huge motivation for me to stay on track. Sometimes it's a struggle, but I think of what my family needs from me, and what I want to give to them and myself, and I get right back on track. Gaining back the weight would be a nightmare. I'm going to be better for Brent."

The days are still hard, and the outlook is uncertain. Getting Brent prepared for school is at least an hour-long routine. It's difficult to see his fanatical interest in football, his desire to play the game, and know that he can't even throw a ball. However, Brent's resourcefulness is an inspiration to everyone around him. For example, Brent himself talked to the coaches of his middle school's football team and convinced them that he should be their mascot. He's already assured of that same position with the high school team when he becomes a freshman next year.

But Brent isn't just a mascot, he's a popular, outgoing, honor-roll student. He has distributed hundreds of small Bibles, which he takes with him wherever he goes. He is, according to his mother, "a beacon in the night, a very special child who has touched many lives."

Faith plays an important part in this story. Initially, Karen felt guilty—she thought she were being punished for something, and that her son's condition was all somehow her fault. This misguided sense of responsibility kept her from seeking any assistance. As her self-esteem improved and she was able to accept the fact that she deserved neither blame nor shame, she reached out and accepted home help. This has lightened her duties, and is another example of how misguided emotions lead to unproductive actions.

A handicap can be a great test of faith, which Karen passed. Angry at first, Karen quickly realized that "this happened for a purpose." In her obese days, Karen didn't want to go anywhere, and felt embarrassed even in church. Now she goes everywhere "with a big smile." Her faith is even stronger, and it helps with her weight maintenance. As she says, "God doesn't go off the wagon, so why should I?"

Although traumatic and difficult situations can confuse us, they can also inspire us. Perhaps Karen needed to gain and lose the 100 pounds to arrive at this point in her life—accepting of her situation; and ready, willing, and able to face whatever comes next.

Rankin's Reminders: Self-Defeat

- Emotions are signs about the meaning of events on our lives. Ideally, those signs are used to guide adaptive action, which will keep life in balance. Too often, however, the emotions themselves take over, and the actions that follow are maladaptive and unproductive. This leads to self-defeat.

For example: A woman wants to lose weight. Her husband say that he'd be so much more attracted to her if she lost the extra pounds. So she gets upset at his comment and uses this anger and resentment to stay fat, thus shooting herself in the foot. Or, a man is diagnosed with cardiac problems: He subsequently panics, goes into denial, and eats his way to even worse health.

- Different emotions arise from different perceptions: Anger arises when you feel unfairly treated by a specific person, frustration occurs when you feel thwarted or blocked by circumstances rather than a person, and guilt stems from the perception that you've violated a moral code.

- Don't act out emotionally. Find ways of managing emotions and devising strategies to solve the challenge that currently faces you. In the above story, Karen was feeling sad, guilty, and overwhelmed. Talking through these problems with others was one way for her to realize that her guilt was misplaced and that help was an acceptable and available alternative.

- Acting emotionally generally means being out of control, and loss of control is the toxic part of stress. So to act emotionally is to make matters worse. Healthy ways of managing emotions include writing in a journal, exercising, meditating, and sharing. (See Chapter 19 for more pointers on managing emotions.)

- Dealing with the situation underlying the emotion is always better than just dealing with the emotion. For example, if you're bingeing and gaining weight because you're in a miserable relationship, you'd be far better off solving the relationship problem rather than trying to assuage anger and resentment by eating.

- Having a plan always restores a sense of control, and devising adaptive strategies to cope with challenges will always make you feel better. Facing a challenge can be rough, but it's almost always better than the alternative.

- When difficult situations arise, remember that their full meaning may take years to become clear. Every challenge comes with benefits, even if they're impossible to see at the time. To paraphrase the Danish philosopher Soren Kierkegaard, life must be lived forward, but it can only be understood backward.

Self-Defeat: Things to Do

1. Listen to your emotions: They're saying something important about your life. For each emotion, there's an underlying challenge.

2. Face challenges head-on. Devise strategies to deal with your problems.

3. Manage your emotions; don't let them manage you.

4. Remember that there's meaning and value in every circumstance, no matter how hard that meaning may be to discern.

5. The best way to manage emotions and devise adaptive strategies is to talk to other supportive people, including health-care professionals.

"If I were to give what I consider the single most useful bit of advice for all humanity, it would be this: Expect trouble as an inevitable part of life, and when it comes, hold your head high, look it squarely in the eye and say, 'I will be bigger than you. You cannot defeat me.'"

— Ann Landers, advice columnist

🌹 🌹 🌹

CHAPTER 11

❋

Weight-Loss Expectations

In the culture in which we live, we've come to demand convenience and immediate results. With weight loss, however, the expectation of a quick and easy transformation is unrealistic and damaging. More reasonable attitudes have to prevail to achieve lasting change.

. . . .

"Pounds in Perspective: Carol Priest"
BY HOWARD J. RANKIN, PH.D.

Although Carol Priest was not overweight as a child, the ingredients were there for a distorted attitude toward food and eating. Carol's father was a product of the Great Depression, and quite authoritarian as well. This meant that mealtimes, always taken at her father's convenience, were tense and unpleasant.

"I was made to feel fortunate to have any food at all, and I was frequently forced to eat everything on my plate, including foods I didn't like. As a result, I was always looking for food and worrying about my next meal. I'd even sneak into the cupboard and steal chocolate chips when no one was looking," Carol admits. "To this day, I have a hard time knowing when I'm satisfied."

When she went away to college and was finally free of parental control, Carol gained weight. "For the first time, I didn't feel guilty about what I ate," Carol says. "No one was there to tell me no." Although she slimmed down when she started dating her future husband, she began to regain the weight just prior to marriage.

Then, in 1989, with her weight hovering around 180 pounds, Carol decided to quit smoking. She recognized the ill effects of her one-pack-a-day habit, and was concerned about secondhand smoke as well as the money she was spending on cigarettes. She found quitting fairly easy. "I was proud of quitting," Carol says, "but I took up eating."

Over the next few years, Carol continued to overeat until she weighed nearly 250 pounds. She had five different sizes of clothes—an escalating wardrobe that was testimony to her increasing weight. On more than one occasion, Carol was asked about her "pregnancy" by people who were merely observing a protruding stomach. Knee, ankle, and back problems prevented her from getting much of an exercise program established, and she was experiencing some symptoms of a cardiovascular condition. She was discouraged. "I was almost at the point where I accepted that I'd be fat forever. I didn't think that I had the determination and persistence to be successful," says Carol.

When Carol joined TOPS, she didn't know what her goal weight would be, because by then she was afraid to get on a scale. It turned out that she needed to lose close to 100 pounds to reach her ideal size. She knew then that she'd have to set about changing her lifestyle.

Carol began by eating more nutritious foods in smaller portions, and eliminating almost all sugar and junk food from her diet. She kept her daily intake of fat under 20 grams, and started walking three miles a day, five days a week. Carol also did two things that are valuable for anyone trying to lose weight: First, she changed her attitude toward food; and second, she took things one day at a time.

In Carol's childhood, hunger meant deprivation, restriction, and abandonment. Hunger encompassed physical *and* emotional emptiness. This legacy continued to haunt her into adulthood and threatened her weight-loss efforts, but she fought back: "I knew that I had to change my thinking about food," she insists. "I had to stop treating each meal or snack as if it were my last, and start thinking of food as fuel for my body."

Knowing that changing her attitude would take some work, Carol got busy. "I surrounded myself with publications on healthy eating, and the more I read, the more I *wanted* to eat sensibly," she says. "I also learned to separate the true feelings of hunger—which actually occurred less and less as I lost the weight—from the emotional hunger pangs, which were my response to feelings of stress, anxiety, or what I call the 'poor-me syndrome.'"

Carol also refused to worry about the amount of weight she had to lose to reach her goal. Instead, she just focused on losing the next pound. Her focus was so intense that she had lost 80 pounds before she realized how close she was to reaching her ideal weight. "I never looked ahead to what was left to lose, only behind at my weekly loss or my loss up to that point," she declares. "When people would ask how many pounds I had left to reach my goal, I had to really stop to figure it out. I had exactly one pound left to go the week before I reached my goal. To me, it was like any other pound—the 1st, the 50th, or the 80th. I weighed in that final week with a four-pound loss."

According to Carol, everyone trying to lose weight has to do the same thing—lose the next pound. Some people have to do this longer than others, but the process is the same for everyone. Using this tactic, Carol lost nearly 90 pounds in 13 months, a weight loss she has maintained for more than 4 years.

* * *

Rankin's Reminders: Weight-Loss Expectations

- It's all too easy to get caught up in a numbers game when you're trying to lose weight. The focus can become almost exclusively on losing pounds rather than changing behavior. Scales are secondary to sensible eating and exercise behavior.

- The scale is an unreliable short-term measure of fat loss. It takes a while, from a few hours to a few days, for fat loss to actually show up on the scale, so weighing yourself every few hours will only lead to discouragement. You can be doing all the right things and burning fat, but that may not be reflected right away. That's why it's advisable to weigh yourself only once a week.

- Unrealistic weight-loss goals can be very discouraging. Following the Federal Trade Commission's crackdown on misleading advertising, ridiculous claims made by weight-loss programs, such as "Lose 20 pounds in a week!" have gone the way of the McLean burger. Nonetheless, many people are still deluded about the rate of weight loss. The truth is that losing two pounds a week requires a 7,000-calorie deficit between energy consumed (food eaten), and energy expended (metabolic rate and exercise).

- The mind works best by focusing on the present. Long-term goals and achievements are often more distracting than motivating, because they can lead to anxiety and discouragement. In the movie *Apollo 13,* which contains many great metaphors about coping, there's a wonderful scene in which Jack Swigert (played by Kevin Bacon) realizes that there's not enough fuel for the spacecraft to return to Earth safely. Commander Jim Lovell (Tom Hanks) then explains that there were a thousand things that had to happen before they reached that point, and that they were currently on number eight. Lovell knew only too well that focusing only on the long-term danger would impact the crew's ability to deal with immediate problems. A tendency to such preoccupation might be natural, but it isn't *adaptive.*

    So remember: When you keep your focus on the next pound, your task is always the same. Moreover, you'll have the satisfaction of reaching short-term goals, and you'll set yourself up for success. When you have manageable short-term weight goals, you can keep your focus on the really important issues—eating and exercise behavior.

Weight-Loss Expectations: Things to Do

1. Set a reasonable weight-loss goal. A reasonable goal is between a half and one and a half pounds per week. That may not sound like a lot, but spread over the course of a year, it equals 25 to 75 pounds.

2. Be *patient.* If you just focus on losing the next pound, you won't get overwhelmed by the daunting task of losing 30, 40, 50, 60, or 100 pounds.

3. Weigh yourself no more frequently than once a week.

4. Concentrate on eating and exercising sensibly, and the scales will follow.

5. Enlist the support of people who will encourage you to reach your short-term goals and focus on the next pound.

🌹

"I've been on a diet for two weeks, and all I've lost is two weeks!"

— Totie Fields, comedienne

🌹 🌹 🌹

CHAPTER 12

❋

Grieving

Food can be such a comfort that it can become a dependable "friend." Giving up that deadly companion is often extraordinarily difficult, but ultimately, it's absolutely crucial.

. . . .

"Saying Good-bye"
BY DOUG ADAMS

When I entered grade school, I was already overweight, and I had to wear "husky" jeans and shirts. I didn't think much of this at the time because I was young. But as I progressed in school, I gained even more weight. I was set apart from the other kids who seemed to enjoy calling me names and making fun of me because of my size. I was the one who was always picked last for sports, and people didn't want to sit next to me. I once went to a neighbor's house, and a child came to the door and said, "Mom, there's a fat boy at the door." On another occasion, I thought that a girl liked me, so we wrote these silly little notes to each other. Then I found out that it was all a joke. When I asked her about it, she told me that I was too fat for anyone to like.

When these sorts of things happened, the only comfort I found was in food. Early on, I discovered that eating made me feel good, like there wasn't anything wrong with me. It comforted my loneliness and hurt, and made me feel as if I was the only thing that mattered. Foods such as cheeseburgers, ice cream, chips, snack cakes, or any type of fried food or dessert were the ones that made me feel the best.

As I entered junior high, I was still gaining weight, because I had now made food my best friend. I did have about three or four school friends, but they didn't offer much support or make me feel as good as fat calories, so I stayed with food. Food and I even played together. We often had sleep-overs when I'd invite food into my room late at night! When I ate, I didn't feel that I was being judged, ridiculed, or criticized. Food was there no matter where I went or what I wanted to do. When I was happy, food was my reward; when I was sad or upset, food was my escape; and when I was nervous, food calmed me down. When I was eating, I was king.

During this time, my mom was a single parent who worked at night. She wasn't home very long after I got home from school before she had to leave, so I was alone a lot. I became more popular with my peers, but I still really didn't have anyone to talk to, hang out with, or call a best friend—except food.

When I got to be about 300 pounds, I started having a hard time breathing because of my weight. I was having difficulty sitting in the little L-shaped desk at school, finding clothes that fit, and even walking. It goes without saying that I couldn't play ball or sports like others did. Basically, I was becoming a couch potato and a hermit, and I had very low self-esteem. I didn't know what to do, so once again, I called my best friend: food.

My family offered me money, new wardrobes, and lots of gifts if I'd just lose 100 pounds, but I wasn't ready to give up my best friend. Everyone seemed to view my weight as a disease or sickness, and felt that I should be able to lose the weight on my own. They didn't understand that I needed someone to show me *how* to let go of my dependence.

When I entered high school, I was already wearing 2X and 3X sizes, and I was well aware that my life was spiraling out of control. I found myself turning to food more and more often—there was no question that it was an addiction. When I graduated from high school, I was at my heaviest ever—350 pounds.

My college experience was very short-lived. I couldn't fit in any of the desks that were available—at best I could prop half of my body in a desk and let the other half hang out in midair. Needless to say, this not only made me physically uncomfortable, but I felt as if everyone was staring at me. I had to schedule all of my classes close to the same building, because if they were across campus from each other, I couldn't get to them in time. It was even difficult for me to walk a flight of stairs without gasping for breath. I was a fish out of water.

I couldn't stand on my feet for long periods of time, so I was really limited as far as employment opportunities went. I had to rely on work in the fast-food or restaurant business, because I didn't have to be standing on my feet all the time—I was able to sit down every two hours for about 15 minutes. This not only affected my attitude, but it also gave me the opportunity to gain more weight. In the restaurants, there was usually no shortage of high calorie, fat-laden food. With my exercise limited because of my ailing feet, ankles, and joints, there was no way I could burn off more than I took in.

As the years went by, I continued to visit my best friend more and more often. I went from job to job, still gaining weight. I went on crash diets to lose the extra pounds and attempt to regain my life, but all I regained was the weight. No matter what I tried, I lost and then I regained what I lost, plus more. I tried a high-protein diet—lost 20, gained 25; a low-carbohydrate diet—lost 35, gained 38; and prescription pills—lost 65, gained 75. If there was a fad diet, I tried it. I even tried starvation—I lost 25 pounds, but gained 40 back when I started eating. I didn't realize that this was killing me—I was just willing to try anything.

My mom and aunt finally introduced me to TOPS, and I started off really well. I made sure I attended the meetings, kept my journal, drank my water, and exercised on a regular basis. I quickly lost 100 pounds, and I was a division winner twice in a row. I kept the 100 pounds off for 11 months, but then I started gaining and gaining until I'd finally gained back everything I'd lost—plus 50 more pounds.

How did it happen? I was a stress eater. I managed a restaurant, and it was a very demanding job. I didn't have any real friends, and I didn't date, which made me feel like an ugly duckling. I was so unhappy. I'd lost all my self-esteem, so once I started to slip and had several weeks in a row where I gained weight, it really upset me. I needed to find other ways of coping with my emotions. But most of all, I just couldn't say good-bye to my friend. That's how I regained 150 pounds.

By the time I was 28, I had developed severe health problems. I'd lost the use of 45 percent of my lungs, and had fluid building up in my feet, ankles, and legs. I could barely walk without gasping for breath, I had high blood pressure, and I couldn't sleep with my mouth closed. I had leaky valves in my heart, which couldn't have helped the heart murmur I was born with. I was also terribly depressed because I couldn't move freely, and I just didn't like myself. I had to have four daily breathing treatments, use an inhaler three times a day, sleep with a CPAP machine (which forces air into your lungs and keeps you breathing while you're asleep), and take 12 pills a day.

When I was 31 and at my highest weight ever—460 pounds—my doctor sent me to see a lung specialist. The specialist tested me and said, "Your weight is crushing your lungs, and it's killing you. If something drastic doesn't happen, and quick, you won't live to see 35." I was finally ready to make a decision: I decided that I wasn't going to live another year in the shape I was in.

If I was going to live, I knew that I had to work at losing weight. With the support of my TOPS chapter, I dedicated myself to exercise, portion control, and drinking plenty of water. Through my efforts, I lost 235 pounds in 18 months, and I saved my own life.

At one stage, I had difficulty just taking care of my day-to-day activities. I couldn't even take a bath because the water and I couldn't fit in the tub at the same time! Now I take long baths. Since I've lost weight, I no longer need pills, a CPAP machine, breathing treatments, or inhalers to get me through the day. Now I'm able to run quarter miles, and I don't have to worry about whether a chair will hold me up or if I'll fit through a certain space. I can buy clothes off the rack, play sports, and hold down a factory job. My doctor, who'd been recommending ankle surgery because of my severe arthritis, has changed his mind, and now no surgery is even being discussed. I can do all the things that a normal person can do. I have a better job, I'm healthier and happier, and I enjoy life to the fullest extent.

I've learned that food doesn't have to be the biggest part of my life. I still feel a void because I've given it up, but I can deal with that now—I'd rather have an occasional longing than a constant depression. I've also learned my limitations. For example, I still can't eat out or attend certain family functions because of the temptation of food. I know that I have to stay away from certain foods in order to maintain and not go on a binge.

Yes, I felt lonely at first, and I thought I wasn't going to make it. When I was really down, I'd call my sister, aunt, friends, and TOPS members. We wrote e-mails and sent notes, and I got an abundance of support and encouragement from them as well as from the TOPS online support groups. Now I have so many people watching me, keeping me in line, and constantly checking up on me that I don't dare regain any weight!

I've realized that food wasn't really my friend, but I still miss it. I've done my best to replace it with real friends and TOPS. I've also coped by being more active, exercising, reading, going on nature walks, and taking time for myself to just get away and focus on my goals. I have a group of TOPS pals online that I know I can turn to when I feel like eating or I'm having problems with my emotions. Sometimes I just need someone to listen.

I've also developed other support groups: people I work with; my church; my sister, Susan; my Aunt Nell; and Grant, who's my best friend. All of these people keep me going and encourage me.

One other thing that keeps me motivated is a picture of myself at my heaviest. It's a constant reminder of where I was, and that I don't want to let myself get back to that point.

It was hard giving up my friend. I still miss her from time to time, but then I remind myself that she wasn't a friend at all. I've regained my life, not my weight, and I'll never go back.

• •

Rankin's Reminders: Grieving

- Personal growth isn't easy. Sometimes it involves uncovering realities that are extremely painful, or giving up relationships or behaviors that seem to be part of your identity. Ending these relationships and behaviors can feel like a psychological amputation.

    Whenever the attempt is made to eliminate a valued behavior, sadness and depression are the natural result. Yet one definition of maturity is the ability to see the destructiveness of a behavior and change it—even if that behavior made you feel great. It's a formidable challenge, but the results are incredibly rewarding.

- In Doug Adams's story, perhaps it would be more accurate to describe food as a lover, rather than just a friend. After all, his relationship with food was certainly passionate and all-consuming. Food seduced him, convinced him of her loyalty, was easily available, and always made him feel good. To his credit, Doug came to realize something that we all have to face at one time or another: Friends and lovers are sometimes mortal enemies in a seductive disguise.

- Having the courage to end a destructive relationship, especially one that has sustained you through good times and bad, is a necessary part of moving on, and the sadness and pain of this loss is best offset by making new friends. That's exactly what Doug did: He replaced his false friend—food—with real, living, loving people.

  So have the courage to let go. Focus on the sly seductiveness of food, rather than its apparent friendship. Make real friends—ones that don't harm you.

- As any addict can tell you, longing never completely disappears. Memories can occur at any moment and throw you into a tailspin. It's precisely at those times that real friends are needed to help keep you grounded and to prevent you from being seduced all over again.

- Don't slide into self-pity—glide into self-improvement.

Grieving: Things to Do

1. On an index card or small piece of paper, write how damaging food really can be. Keep the card with you at all times.

2. Identify real friends who can be contacted when you're in withdrawal over the loss of your beloved food.

3. As with every loss, the pain fades over time. The longer you can

go without rekindling your emotional relationship with food, the better off you'll be.

4. Practice throwing your favorite food away.

5. Identify others with whom you can share feelings and attitudes about food. Replace food with real friends.

"The only cure for grief is action."

— George Henry Lewes, philosopher

CHAPTER 13

❊

Excuses

We all make excuses. They magically pop into our heads at exactly the right time and promise to bail us out of those actions we really don't want to take. It's not having the excuse that's important, it's how we challenge the excuses once they mysteriously appear in our consciousness.

• •

"Fooling Yourself: Threasa Schwegman"
BY HOWARD J. RANKIN, PH.D.

Threasa was never overweight as a child or teen. She weighed 120 pounds when she got married in 1974, and gradual weight gain followed. After the birth of her son in 1976, she decided to be a stay-at-home mom. "I think the soap operas and too much leisure time got the best of me. *Days of Our Lives* and a bag of chips was the daily norm!" she says.

After the birth of her second child seven years later, Threasa's weight exceeded 150 pounds. It was time to do something, so she "crash dieted," living mostly on diet soda and light snacks, dropping 50 pounds in one summer. At about the same time, she was diagnosed with rheumatoid arthritis. It was hard to know whether the arthritis or the dieting was causing the weight loss. Either way, she was glad she was losing weight, even when her doctors started expressing deep concern that she'd lost too much. She began taking medications for the arthritis and slowly began to gain weight again. Over the next 19 years, she gained all her weight back, plus about 40 more pounds. She was near 190 when she finally decided to join TOPS.

Threasa now knows that extreme diets can be very harmful. "I'll always believe that my unhealthy dieting put a severe strain on my immune system, which may have triggered the rheumatoid arthritis that I now live with," she says.

Threasa was introduced to a lady in her town who also had arthritis. They shared information about different doctors and various medications that they were each taking. "One day I casually mentioned to her that I knew I'd feel much better if I could just lose some weight. Wow! It was like a lightbulb lit up her face," says Threasa. "She proceeded to tell me that she was the TOPS leader in our town, and she invited me to come to a meeting."

Threasa put off going to a meeting for several months before finally deciding she really should check it out. Part of her didn't want to make the effort to lose the weight, and part of her didn't want to have to make a commitment to a group. When she did finally attend, however, she instantly changed her mind.

"I attended my first meeting and decided on the spot to commit to this program. My doctor and I set a weight-loss goal of 50 pounds, which I reached in 13 months," says Threasa. "All my heartfelt thanks go to my husband for his support at home, but I simply wouldn't have had the motivation to lose those 50 pounds without the encouragement of all my TOPS friends!"

Threasa looks back at the excuses she made to avoid joining the TOPS group and smiles. As a testimony to these rationalizations, Threasa created a list of ten common excuses for not joining a TOPS group, and why they just don't hold water. So here they are:

Threasa Schwegman's Top Ten Reasons for Not Joining TOPS
(and Why She's So Glad She Did)

1. *I'm just not a "meeting" person.*

    I could tell from the very first night I went that
    TOPS meetings would not only be fun, but very organized
    and informative. The programs are always something to
    look forward to—anything from women's health issues,
    to exercise, to dressing in order to look slimmer.

2. *I don't want to diet. Diets don't work for me.*

    I've dieted before, and it didn't work. When I lost
    the 50 pounds after my daughter was born, I did it by
    living on diet soda and popcorn. I'm convinced that
    this compromised my immune system, which triggered
    my arthritis. I learned from TOPS that I could lose
    weight by changing my lifestyle. I had 20 years of poor
    eating and exercise habits that had to be changed.

3. *I hate exercising!*

    The summer before I joined TOPS, I went with
    my daughter to her freshman orientation at college.
    There were a lot of walking tours, and I found myself
    having to stop several times just to catch my breath. I
    knew something had to be done. Soon after joining
    TOPS, I began to walk, just 10 to 15 minutes at a
    time. I remember my legs tingling at first—a sure sign
    that I was out of shape!

    Gradually, however, I worked myself up to two
    miles a day, and now I actually look forward to it!
    Sometimes I'll get up early in the morning and walk
    while the sun rises, and other times stepping out in the
    late afternoon helps me clear my head after a busy day.
    On the country road where I walk, I can experience
    the beauty of nature that I might otherwise pass by.

4. *I take medication that causes weight gain, so I probably won't be able to lose anything.*

    Nope, you can't use that excuse. I tried to, but then I talked to my TOPS leader. She takes the same medication that I do, and she managed to lose weight. Besides that, when the doctor told me about possible weight gain from my medication, he probably meant 5 or 10 pounds, not 50! I still take the same medication, but since my weight loss, I hardly ever experience arthritic pain anymore.

5. *I'm just not ready to make a commitment.*

    Why not? When I joined TOPS, I'd just put my last child in college, and I decided it was time to do something for me. So I joined the Tuesday after September 11, 2001. That event was a wake-up call that life is very short, and you need to do what you can to make the best of every day—including keeping yourself healthy.

6. *I love to eat. It's my only source of entertainment.*

    My husband and I still love to eat out, but most restaurants offer low-fat entrees, and there are so many healthy choices I can make. I've never felt deprived on the TOPS program. I just eat more sensibly. I can even go to McDonald's and have a Fruit 'n Yogurt Parfait for only 280 calories and 4 grams of fat (without granola).

7. *I just can't drink all that water.*

    You need water! My skin was very dry from the effects of my arthritis medication, but after increasing the amount of water I drank, I soon began to notice a change. Water really does help with those hunger pangs—and think of the money you'll save on sodas!

8. *I'm shy. I don't think I want to get up and share my feelings in front of a group.*

    I was made to feel so welcome and at ease in front of my TOPS chapter. Typically, we discuss magazine articles or something that's of interest to us all.

9. *I won't know anyone there.*

    Even though I didn't know many of the people in my group, that all soon changed. Everyone was so kind and friendly. The support I received with cards, e-mails, and phone calls has made all the difference. Even though we all come from different backgrounds and age groups, we all share common issues related to our weight. Who could help me more than someone who's going through the same thing that I am?

10. *I'm afraid I won't be able to lose the weight. I've tried too many times before, and I'll probably fail this time, too.*

    I mentioned the word *commitment* before. That's what it's all about. I never refer to TOPS as a diet, it's a healthy lifestyle change. I've done away with a lot of bad habits, and I know what it takes to keep the weight off. I can *never* eat the way I did again!

    My goal was to lose one pound a week, which would mean about 50 pounds in a year. Surely I could do that! Sometimes I'd achieve my short-term goal of a pound a week, and sometimes I wouldn't, but my TOPS friends kept on encouraging me even when I gained (and we all have weeks like that sometimes). Just keep on track, stay focused on your goals, and make each day a new day. And be consistent! There's a saying that "slow and steady wins the race." That has become my motto over the last year, so even if it's a quarter-pound loss, I count my blessings because they all add up.

● ●

Rankin's Reminders: Excuses

- There are thousands of excuses that can justify the avoidance of the weight-loss issue. Of course, these excuses are not valid justifications at all—just rationalizations to avoid the effort involved in losing weight and keeping it off. Threasa's excuses had to do with the avoidance of actually attending a group, but here are some other classic examples.

   1. *Now is not the right time. I have too much to do, the planets aren't properly aligned, my horoscope is against it, and it's a month with a vowel in it.*

       You need to wake up to the fact that there's never a "right time." If you wait for everything to be perfect, it will never happen. Besides, you need to overcome those perfectionist tendencies or they'll set you up for failure.

   2. *I can't exercise because my knees hurt, and without being able to exercise, there's no point in trying to lose weight.*

       Hello! Your knees hurt because you're overweight, and there's something seriously wrong with your thinking if you're using excess weight as an excuse to not lose weight! There are many exercises that can be done that don't stress knees, joints, or other parts of the anatomy that might be under duress. Even if you're paralyzed, you can eat healthier and lose weight. I know several people who are wheelchair-bound, and they do exercises from their wheelchairs and manage to lose weight. (Remember Marie Wagner from Chapter 6?) If you're upright, you can burn calories—and I'll bet you can walk when you're shopping.

       At a recent State Recognition Day, I met two women who told me how difficult if was for them to move, let alone exercise. Later that evening, there was a handsome Elvis impersonator as the main entertainment. When he seductively invited members of the audience onstage, these two sup- posedly immobile ladies rushed up as if they'd been shot out of a cannon! I suppose it all comes down to what motivates you.

3. *Eating right and exercising is expensive, and I can't afford it right now.*

Regrettably, the cost of healthy food *is* higher than the cost of junk food, and exercise does involve an investment in a good pair of walking shoes. However, these costs are minimal compared to the health-care expenses involved in treating respiratory and cardiac conditions, joint problems, and diabetes—not to mention the personal cost of low self-esteem.

4. *I have a family to look after, and they come first.*

If you've ever been in an airplane, you've been told that in the event of an emergency, the oxygen masks will deploy—and you're instructed to give yourself oxygen *before* helping children or others who depend on you. Why? Because you're no use to anyone if you can't breathe! Families need par- ents who are in optimal physical and mental health. If you're miserable because of excess weight, if moving around is difficult, or if you're depressed and grouchy or just downright antisocial, then your family isn't going to benefit. Stop using your loved ones as an excuse, and get in shape for them.

5. *I'm genetically predisposed to being heavy, so there's nothing I can do about it.*

It sounds as if you're also genetically prone to making excuses. But even if you really are genetically programmed to being overweight, there's *always* something you can do about it. There are many normal-weight people who have a genetic predisposition to being overweight, but they eat and exercise in a way that nullifies this predisposition. A genetic disposition isn't a death sentence—it's an invitation to lead a healthy lifestyle.

6. *I'm not so bad—other people are far worse off than me.*

    With this type of thinking, you'll sink to the lowest level. If you have to compare yourself with others, compare yourself to those functioning at a higher level—not a lower one. Yes, there are always people worse off than you, but I guarantee that you really wouldn't want to be living their lives. So be careful what you wish for: This excuse will only make you worse off.

7. *I'm really just big-boned, not overweight.*

    Yes, your main problem is that you are too short for your weight. Practice good height management and you should be absolutely fine! You might consider joining the support group Gain Height Sensibly.

8. *I'm still young. I can lose weight when I'm a little older.*

    In one of the more compelling health-related statistics, a recent study showed that 100 percent of people do get older. But seriously, the best time to gain control of your weight is when you're young. It's much more difficult to do as you get older, when metabolism, energy, and mobility slow down.

9. *This lifestyle-change stuff is too much effort. I'll wait for the magic pill.*

    I'm afraid you can't bank on a magic pill being invented anytime soon. And if there were one, it probably wouldn't make that much difference. Stop medicalizing everything, and appreciate the enormous impact of culture: We live in a fat society that makes normal people overweight! The vast majority of overweight Americans don't have a genetic predisposition to obesity—they just eat too much and exercise too little—so a fat pill is probably not going to make a whole lot of difference.

If you want more evidence of the myths of medicalization, consider gastric-bypass surgery. People who have undergone this surgery will tell you that it's *not* a quick fix, and it's useless without lifestyle change.

10. *Being fat isn't bad for you. All this doom and gloom about excess weight is a medical conspiracy put out by doctors, hospitals, and pharmaceutical companies to scare people and increase business.*
     Yeah, and Santa Claus is in the CIA.

Excuses: Things to Do

1. The mind is really ingenious in creating instant rationalizations that can plant doubt in even the strongest person. Consider this one: *I've been walking in the mall for an hour and a half. I bet my blood sugar is dangerously low by now. If I don't get some ice cream in me soon, I might faint and cause great embarrassment right here in front of all these shoppers!* If you do have a "brainstorm" like this one, try sharing it with someone else before acting out on it, or just keep walking and see if you can find the flaws in it. (If you can't, you're in big trouble!)

2. The best way to deal with rationalizations is to not deviate from your plans unless you absolutely have to. And always try to consider the potential effects of your choices before acting out.

3. Think of the people who are worse off than you. You're lucky you can do all the things that you can!

4. Keep a list of people you can call when motivation is wavering and excuses are jumping around in your head like popcorn in a popper.

5. Write down ten excuses to avoid weight loss with your buddies and discuss them. You could even have a contest called "Lamest Excuses of the Year."

"The best measure of a man's honesty isn't his income tax return.
It's the zero adjust on his bathroom scale."

— Arthur C. Clarke, author

CHAPTER 14

❀

Spirituality

One of the themes of this book is that isolation is unproductive and that positive relationships can transform your life. Tammy Hopkins reminds us that those relationships begin with a connection to a higher power.

· ·

"A Force That's Bigger Than I Am"
BY TAMMY HOPKINS

Even as a child, I was overweight. In the second grade, a girl slapped me while I was sitting on the school bus. She said I was fat and couldn't sit with her. I was constantly picked on, I was always chosen last to play sports, and I had very few friends, so I learned to hide inside myself. The truth is, I didn't need other people to tear me down—I did enough of that all by myself.

I started dieting in my teenage years. During high school, I drank diet root beer mixed with powdered Slim-Fast. I also took Vivarin to keep up my energy. Later I tried liquid diets; low-carb diets; pills; a banana-only diet; high-protein diets; and yes, even starvation. I failed again and again. I was too hard on myself, and I couldn't stick with these diets. Every time

I tried, I just put more weight on. I decided that diets don't work, so I'd just have to live the way that I am. I became very absorbed in my own self-pity and negativity.

In December of 1997, God began dealing with my heart. He was the only one who knew how I felt about myself. During one church service, the preacher said, "If you don't love *yourself,* how can you love God?" I remember crying, and I started praying, asking God for help. I hated that I was overweight, and I hated that I was too weak to change myself. I had a hard time believing that my husband loved me, because all I could see in myself was a fat, incompetent, shy person.

I knew I couldn't do it alone. I'd tried many times before, but I always failed. So this time I prayed daily for the strength and courage to face my weight problem. I hadn't ever asked for anything with such passion before. I'd actually felt that I was too fat to do anything for God, so why should He want to help me? But God answered my prayers through a lady at church named Lois.

It was very hard to accept Lois's advice and go to her TOPS chapter in Joshua, Texas. I didn't want to face a group of people and admit that I was overweight. However, on January 12, 1998, with shaky legs and sweaty palms, I walked a long sidewalk up to the double doors of the church where the meeting was held. On the other side of the threshold stood smiling ladies, full of hugs. They encouraged me to weigh in. I weighed 276 pounds. I dreaded the weigh-in, but the scales were in a closed room, with just two people to record the information. The weight recorder was very friendly, and she was discreet with everyone's private information.

It didn't take long for me to realize that these women were just like me, stuck in the same situation I was in. They had the same sad scars on their hearts, and the same hopes and fears. Of course there was a shining star, the one who'd already reached her goal. Her name was Hazel, and she had been a KOPS member for four years.

That night, I thanked God and promised myself that I wasn't going to quit. I had no more excuses. God can do all things, and I'd asked him for help. He gave me the answer I needed in TOPS. What could stop me know?

One of the most important things I did was change my "I can't" attitude into an "I can" one. I recognized that the choice was mine, and I believed it! Every week, without fail, I went to TOPS. They taught me how to keep food and walking charts. They gave me advice to help me reach my goal and taught me about nutrition, exercise, motivation, and having a positive attitude. They also coaxed me into making some presentations to the group, which helped me get out of my comfort zone, interact with new people, and learn to accept compliments.

My doctor advised me to count calories. We set a goal of about 1,000 calories a day, and I started planning my meals in a way that I'd never done before. It became a game. I found many food combinations that I liked, and I discovered that I could eat quite a lot for 1,000 calories. I also realized how many calories I was consuming before: I'd often eat close to 2,000 calories in one sitting—a Quarter-Pounder with cheese, large fries, and a Coke, topped off with a vanilla ice-cream cone.

I exchanged red meat for chicken, ham, and lean pork. I chose carrots, popcorn, and apples instead of French fries and potato chips, and I enjoyed frozen yogurt instead of ice cream. I also learned that potatoes have flavor without being loaded with sour cream, cheese, bacon, and butter. To top it all off, I completely eliminated sodas. I used to drink a 44-ounce fountain soda with my lunch—that's 410 calories. Besides, I found that drinking water could help me lose weight faster.

I began trying more forms of exercise, the first of which was walking. At first it was very difficult, as I wasn't used to any exercise; I was happy to walk a mile. I had 276 pounds on my 5'5" frame, so my legs ached at night. I took Tylenol and prayed that I'd be able to do better tomorrow. Eventually, I did a lot of walking—about 25 to 30 miles a week. If I had a few extra minutes in the day, I'd jog in place or touch my toes, whatever I could do to raise my heart rate. I started earning TOPS walking and weight-loss charms, which are awarded for reaching certain goals. Eventually, I had so many charms on my bracelet that I chimed with each stride.

With all of these new habits, the weight just fell off. I lost 115 pounds the first year and never gained any back. Now I've lost more than 130 pounds, and I have my TOPS friends to thank for keeping me in line. Of course, I did have rough days—we all do. At times I wanted to quit. But I really valued my program, so every morning I'd wake up and recommit to it. I didn't want to take anything for granted.

I learned not to make excuses. If I couldn't walk, I'd find another way to get exercise. When chocolate began to call me in the middle of the night, I stopped buying it. I didn't deprive my husband and kids of snacks, I simply bought the ones they liked but I didn't. I had to keep reminding myself, *You're worth it!*

Each time I lost another 12 pounds, I'd reward myself with a new dress in my new size. That was a great motivator for me. My greatest inspiration, however, came from my husband and my daughter, Kendra. Kendra was thrilled that she could put her arms around me, and she also enjoyed taking long walks and playing basketball with me. She didn't even complain about all of the chicken I was feeding her! I only wish I could have some of those overweight years back to play with her the way I can now.

My husband of 17 years, Ken, never complained about my weight. When we married, I was a size 20, but I progressed to a 28. Now, he's extremely proud of me, and what a way to add that extra spark to your marriage! I like all of the extra attention and compliments he gives me. Now, we spend quality time together, taking walks or talking—anything other than just sitting mindlessly in front of the television.

I've changed as much on the inside as I have on the outside. I have a positive, fun-loving attitude now. I'm not afraid to try new things. I now sing in front of the whole church congregation, and I can speak to large groups of people—things I would have never done in the past. I'm living life to the fullest.

I no longer hide behind myself; instead, I look to see how I can help others. I want to hug the people who are like I used to be and tell them that they can do it! That's why I'm still active in TOPS—to give back some of what TOPS has given to me. I talk to as many people as I can and encourage them to make a real commitment to their health.

I've won several major awards, including being the TOPS Charm and Beauty contest runner-up in 2002 in Colorado Springs. From 1991 until 1992, my husband and I lived there, but at the time, I wasn't able to enjoy the outdoors because I weighed too much. So, when I returned in 2002, I was much more active and able to enjoy many of the scenic wonders that the area had to offer. For example, I climbed several hundred steps at Seven Falls and never broke a sweat. I could even see my feet on the way down! To make it perfect, my husband was there to share in my triumph.

In January of 2002, I ran a marathon at Walt Disney World in Orlando. It was unreal. I chose to do the leukemia marathon because I wanted to help a worthy cause. I felt as if I were giving back some of what was given to me—life. Finishing the marathon was exhilarating. I cried because of the pain, but also because of the feeling of happiness that filled me completely. The experience reinforced the idea that I can do anything if I step outside myself and appreciate the awesome force of a higher power.

● ●

Rankin's Reminders: Spirituality

- The hallmark of spirituality is the recognition that there are greater and more important cosmic forces than your ego. This recognition is as empowering as it is humbling, because it provides security, courage, and strength to deal with life's challenges.

- Spirituality will get you away from self-absorption and put your life into proper perspective, because it encourages you to find meaning in your actions and in life in general. This is important because weight loss doesn't happen in a vacuum, it has deep personal meaning—and awareness of meaning will enhance whatever you attempt, including weight loss.

- Spirituality is not a cop-out. Turning your life over to a higher power doesn't mean that you no longer take responsibility, quite the contrary. Spirituality makes you *more* responsible by recognizing your connection to others and accountability to your God. It also provides the confidence to take effective action by instilling faith.

- Spirituality is manifested in managing your own life effectively and in helping others.

- Your connection with your higher power needs constant attention.

Spirituality: Things to Do

1. Be aware that as an individual, you're a very small part of the universe.

2. Pray, meditate, or do whatever you need to do to stay mindful and connected to your higher power.

3. Within reasonable limits of your resources, find ways of helping others. Helping others is humility in action.

4. Observe your behavior from others' perspectives. Ask for feedback and reality checks on your actions.

5. Don't be defensive or judgmental.

🌹

The next section of this book, Part III, contains stories that identify 12 specific skills and behaviors that are essential for weight loss and personal transformation.

🌹

*"When an objective is meaningful, joy is
a natural consequence of its pursuit."*

— Allen Wiesen, psychologist

PART III

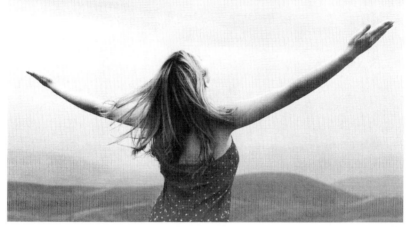

Skills

CHAPTER 15

❋

Patience

We've all heard the saying "Patience is a virtue." Well, in our society, patience is a rapidly disappearing trait. One common mistake that we sometimes make when trying to lose weight quickly is to radically change our lifestyle all at once. This is a setup for failure.

. . . .

"Do One Thing: Donna Simoneaux"
BY HOWARD J. RANKIN, PH.D.

Donna Simoneaux was in the grocery store. She'd just put a candy bar into her cart when she heard a stranger's voice.

"You don't need that candy bar!" said a man who was buying a pack of cigarettes. Obviously he was passing judgment on Donna's 5'2", 211-pound frame.

Donna was embarrassed and mad. *You're one to talk,* she thought as she left the store. *You're creating secondhand smoke and harming others. At least I'm just hurting myself.*

Sometimes simply hearing yourself think can lead to important insights, and later that day, Donna realized the implications of her thoughts:

She had rationalized that it was acceptable to hurt herself. "But it's not okay for me to mistreat myself," Donna reflects. "And besides, I *wasn't* just hurting myself—I was hurting my family, too." That realization was enough for Donna to take action.

Still, when Donna joined TOPS, she wasn't sure that she was ready to begin a weight-loss program. "I didn't really want to join, but three of my friends were going to start attending meetings, and I didn't want to pass up the opportunity to get involved with people I knew—I didn't have the guts to go alone," she explains.

"Now, in my mind, I'd always imagined that joining TOPS would be my last resort for successful weight loss," says Donna. "I used to say that if all else failed, then I'd try TOPS and be able to succeed. I just figured that when I joined, I'd be ready to lose weight. I'm not sure why I felt that way. It may have been that I'd heard of other people's successes and figured that if they could do it, I could, too. So I *had* to do something to make this program work."

Then, when Donna's mother died just six weeks after being diagnosed with stomach cancer, she found even more motivation to lose the weight for good. Donna's mom had been heavily involved in her church and had helped many people. At her funeral, the church was packed, and the wonderful service with a full choir lasted two hours. "I realized how many people Mom had touched, and I was really moved," Donna recalls. "But then I realized that *I* hadn't touched anybody." The idea that she could positively influence people by being a role model fueled Donna's determination even more. "Weight was my arena. I knew about it, and I felt that I could make a difference," she says.

Donna faced many challenges on the path to weight loss: a busy work schedule, mothering two children, a thyroid problem, and a Cajun culture that thrives on desserts and foods cooked in flour and heavy oil, to name a few. After her medical condition was relieved by the removal of her thyroid, her most difficult challenge became trying to change a lifetime pattern of eating habits while continuing to live her everyday life.

"I was still reeling from grief at losing my mother, and I knew that I didn't want to feel deprived," Donna explains. "I needed to do something to make a difference without causing too much of a disruption. I'd cut out sugary sodas before, so that wasn't a very difficult change for me. Since I never liked the aftertaste of diet drinks, I eliminated all soft drinks from my diet during my first week with TOPS, drinking water instead."

After she replaced sodas with water, Donna switched to fat-free snacks. "I wasn't going to starve myself—I still wanted treats now and then. Eliminating them entirely would've left me feeling sorry for myself, and that wouldn't have boded well for long-term weight loss. The first snack to change was potato chips: Instead of regular chips, I tried pretzels, Bugles, Air Crisps, and finally, Baked Lay's. I'm a person who doesn't like a whole lot of change at one time, so when I found something that I liked, I stayed with it until I grew tired of it."

Just making these minor changes resulted in some weight loss. Desserts were the next to go, and then grilled chicken replaced hamburger meat. Dietary modifications were made every two to three weeks, which gave new behaviors a chance to become established habits before additional changes were made.

Eventually Donna switched to smaller plates to cut back on portion size, and she eliminated second helpings. She read nutrition labels to be sure that she never ate anything that was more than 30-percent fat—that way, she could be sure that her overall fat intake was under that level. She describes her progress as gradual: "At first, when I went to a fast-food restaurant, I'd order the small fries along with the grilled-chicken sandwich, opting for the smaller portion rather than depriving myself of something that I enjoyed. After a time, the fries became something that I could do without, so in order to keep losing weight, I stopped ordering them. Then I stopped going to fast-food restaurants altogether, preferring to frequent a sit-down restaurant where I could make better choices and eat a decent meal, or fixing a turkey sandwich to bring on the road."

In keeping with her progressive approach, Donna began to exercise. "When I started, I didn't want to get up any earlier in the morning, because I felt that I needed all the sleep I could get—I was always so tired. So I exercised in the afternoon." She set a fairly modest goal of walking one mile in the afternoon, and she gradually increased her routine to up to four miles a day. "I knew from past experience that it takes two to three weeks of doing something before you should add to it," Donna says, "so I made changes in my exercise program on a scheduled basis. Eventually I started adding morning exercise to my routine. I only got up a few minutes earlier, eliminating the two extra snooze periods I usually took after my alarm clock went off. I soon realized that I felt better when I woke up without snoozing, so it was easier to get up a little earlier and add more time to my morning workout. It also made me feel a whole lot better during the day."

Donna developed a strategy for increasing the amount of time she spent exercising. "I love to read, and I noticed that I was much more motivated to keep walking when I was reading. So I set a rule for myself that I could only read while I was working out. Whenever I was reading something really good and didn't want to stop, I'd add a few minutes to the treadmill so that I could finish that part of the book. This practice eventually got me walking 60 minutes a day with 5-minute warm-up and cooldown periods, and it motivated me to get up earlier in order to be able to complete my routine."

TOPS meetings also played a big role in keeping Donna inspired. At TOPS there were many women who had known Donna's mother, and they were sympathetic toward Donna and gave her a lot of hugs. Donna felt that these people were a direct connection to her mom. "People would say, 'Your mom would be so proud of you.' I needed that," she says. Donna also engaged in healthy competition with her friend and fellow TOPS member Norma. Each week they'd vie to see who had the biggest weight loss. Moreover, both Norma and Donna were inspired by Sandy Callais (whose story is featured in this book), who was on her way to losing 90 pounds.

The first 50 of Donna's 75-pound weight loss came off in about 18 months, and it took her another year to finally reach her goal weight. Two thoughts helped her through the inevitable temptations: When she wanted something, she asked herself, *Is it worth it?* and *Will it result in a gain?* "I've learned to listen to my body and go with what's manageable," she says.

After a while, Donna began to see food in a different light. "I had to change my attitude toward food. Fat was my proclaimed enemy, so to reduce the amount of fat in my diet, I needed to change the way I thought about fried foods, such as doughnuts—a particular vice of mine. I'd envision a doughnut being dunked in hot oil, soaking up all that grease. Then I'd think about what happens to the oil when it cools. I'd visualize the doughnut cooling and that soaked-up oil coagulating. Now when I look at a doughnut—most of the time, anyway—I no longer see a sweet, tempting treat, but a congealed lump of lard. It's not quite so tempting when I imagine it this way!" Donna exclaims.

Today, Donna is a chapter leader, and she's making a difference in people's lives. She writes notes of encouragement to at least ten TOPS members every week, and she has found meaning in her life by reaching out and touching people, just like her mother did.

"I've seen a number of people lose weight quickly by making a lot of changes immediately. Unfortunately, it's really difficult to maintain a whole set of new healthy habits at once, and slipping up can lead to discouragement and weight gain. But I know that this won't be the case with me. My patient approach means that there are still a number of things I can change if I choose to, sort of a 'last resort'—like joining TOPS in the first place."

- -

Rankin's Reminders: Patience

When it comes to lifestyle modification, the golden rule is to *focus on changing one behavior at a time.* Unfortunately, many people don't know this, so their attempts to change habits are almost doomed from the start.

There are several reasons why patience is key:

- It establishes realistic expectations. Most of us dramatically underestimate the difficulty of changing behaviors, especially ones as complicated as eating and exercising. By breaking a behavior down into smaller components, the scope of what's required to effect a lifestyle change becomes more realistic.

- It ensures focus. Energy is directed to just one area, rather than being dispersed into many different places. This makes changing behavior more manageable and prevents feelings of being overwhelmed, which are common at the beginning of any weight-loss attempt.

- A patient technique gives a sense of building up to a program rationally step-by-step, rather than just taking a shotgun approach. It requires people to *think* about each behavior that needs to be changed, and it helps to prioritize these changes.

- People learn best by trial-and-success, and achieving small gains helps build confidence and hope. Patiently focusing on one behavior at a time also makes it easier to monitor progress and determine success.

- Over time, original changes can be modified to fine-tune your program. For example, Donna went from eating burgers and fries at fast-food restaurants, to switching to chicken sandwiches, to eliminating the fries, to avoiding fast food altogether.

Patience: Things to Do

1. Identify five behaviors that need to be changed for you to meet your goals. For example:

   - Drink water instead of soda.

   - Limit fat intake to less than 30 percent of total calories consumed.

   - Skip dessert.

   - Add or increase exercise.

   - Eliminate junk food.

2. Choose one new behavior from your list to change, and faithfully practice it for at least a week—until you feel you've mastered it. Then add another behavior change, and so on.

3. Monitor progress by writing your performance down in a journal.

4. Identify people who can help you successfully make these changes. Enlist their support by telling them how they can assist you.

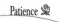

5. When you've mastered your first list of five behaviors, compile another one.

"Have patience with all things, but chiefly have patience with yourself. Do not lose courage in considering you own imperfections, but instantly set about remedying them—every day begin the task anew."

— Saint Francis de Sales

CHAPTER 16

❊

Visualization

In this story of tragedy and courage, Bonnie Cesana tells how she transformed her life by using the power of visualization to overcome grief, cancer, and obesity.

. . . .

"Seeing Is Believing: Bonnie Cesana"
BY HOWARD J. RANKIN, PH.D.

Food and eating were always at the center of social activity in Bonnie Cesana's household. Growing up in a home where food meant love, it wasn't surprising that most of her family was overweight. Despite a great early childhood (or perhaps *because* of it), Bonnie was no exception.

Tragedy first struck when Bonnie was 12 years old. One day when she returned home from school, she was met at the door by a neighbor who told her that her father was ill and had been taken to the hospital. He never returned, having died of a heart attack at the age of 57.

"The earth stopped," says Bonnie. Perhaps that's why she was more than a little overweight by the time she was a sophomore in high school: Standing 5'5", she weighed 170 pounds. But luckily, she wasn't there for long. She found a summer child-care job that she loved, and it kept her active and away from the kitchen. She quickly lost 30 pounds—a loss that she maintained through her college years and into her early married life.

But three pregnancies in less than five years added an extra 40 pounds, and by the time Bonnie's mother came to live with her several years later, another 25 had crept on. Her mother had Alzheimer's disease, and having her at home—along with three kids—was difficult. So Bonnie attempted to keep her mom grounded through familiar routines, many of which were centered around cooking and the kitchen. In this family's culture, calories and closeness were intimately related. Finally, the time came when her mother could no longer be cared for at home.

When her last child started college, Bonnie was finally relieved of her role as caregiver. Her kids were all doing well—Martin was at West Point, Jennifer was attending New York Medical College, and Jessica was studying music at Ithaca College. The business Bonnie and her husband had started in 1973 was doing well, and life was good.

At about this same time, Bonnie took up a new sport. Although she'd always been an avid walker and cross-country skier, one of her daughters encouraged her to try Alpine skiing, and Bonnie, at the age of 46, loved it. Encouraged by the joy and exhilaration of this new activity, and with a renewed focus on healthier eating, she lost about 50 pounds.

Yet in spite of her efforts, Bonnie was still 30 pounds overweight. "I was always doing just enough to keep off the really high weight, but never doing enough to get down to where I needed be," says Bonnie. "Typically, I'd diet from January through March, but then resume old habits and regain whatever weight I'd lost, plus a few pounds more. The following January I'd repeat the process. I never quite got weight control."

This cycle was disrupted when, for the second time in her life, Bonnie's world stopped turning. One morning the Cesanas got a call. It started with four words that every parent dreads: "There's been an accident." Their son, Martin, a captain in the Army and a trainer in the desert-warfare program at Fort Irwin in California, had been critically injured during maneuvers.

A sudden dust storm had temporarily created havoc, and during the chaos, a tank had run into Martin's Humvee. Martin was evacuated by helicopter to the hospital. Immediately, Bonnie and her husband set out for

California, but they were too late. By the time they got there, Martin was dead. A beloved son, brother, colleague, and friend was lost forever.

In the following months, Bonnie and her family looked at the world through a veil of tears. Grieving over the loss of Martin, they asked a thousand times, "Why?" There was no answer, only silence. They just couldn't believe it. "His clothes, motorcycles, snowboards, and car were returned to us. These daily reminders of the son we lost intensified our grief, and yet we couldn't bear to part with his possessions," says Bonnie. The memory of Martin's last phone call echoed through Bonnie's mind, and a Mother's Day card with photographs, sent by her son before the accident, arrived in the mail. Profound grief enveloped the family, then anger. What would have been Martin's 30th birthday passed in sorrow, as did the first Christmas without him.

Martin had inherited his family's love of food, and even as a young boy, he enjoyed cooking and baking. This passion continued through adulthood, and at Fort Irwin, Martin had a reputation in his unit as a great cook. Out in the field, he'd make gourmet meals in his black cast-iron Dutch oven. Now, in memory of his talent, there's a place out in the desert next to a cliff called Marty's Kitchen, dedicated by friends, family, and colleagues who gather there to honor him. On a pedestal stands his Dutch oven, and a brass plaque mounted on the rock behind it bears these words: "His cooking satisfied our hunger, his friendship satisfied our spirits."

At this point in Bonnie's life, losing weight wasn't important. Getting through each day and getting some sleep each night was now her main goal. Grief-stricken, Bonnie gained more than 30 pounds in the following year, reaching her all-time heaviest: 230 pounds.

It was then, in April of 1997, 11 months after Martin's death, that Bonnie joined TOPS. "I just loved the group support," she says. "It's so much easier losing weight when you're not alone. I loved the fact that if I had a problem, I had a group of people to bounce ideas off. Left to my own devices, I'd allow the problems to wear me down."

In her first year, Bonnie lost 38 pounds. The next year she was able to drop another 13, but it was more difficult. Bonnie often doubled her exercise from one to two hours a day, but progress was still slow. By April of 2000, she had lost 60 pounds and had 15 more to go. She was determined to achieve her goal within the next nine months, a personal celebration of the millennium.

"I realized that I needed to become more vigilant, to really focus," Bonnie admits. "My pattern was to be good for a while, but then slip enough to slow my progress. I knew the right thing to do, but when there was a plate of my favorite food in front of me, it was hard to resist."

The technique that Bonnie used to regain focus was *visualization*. "I'd used this technique when learning to ski, and again a few years later when learning to snowboard," she says. "By taking time at night to visualize the position of my body, I internalized what the instructor had taught me during the day. It helped me to be more successful the next time I was actually on the slopes.

"I also read about this technique in a study comparing three groups of basketball players. Group A practiced free-throw shots as usual, while Group B spent twice as much time as the first group making the shots. Group C practiced the same amount as the first group, but each individual in this group spent extra time visualizing the procedure by which successful free-throw shots were made," Bonnie explains. "After some weeks, the three groups were compared. Group A improved the least, while Group C improved almost as much as Group B. This proves that visualization definitely helps boost performance. So I decided to apply this concept to weight loss."

Each day Bonnie spent a few minutes visualizing weight-loss success. The first thing she imagined was wearing pretty clothes. "I hadn't bought many clothes, certainly not pretty ones, since I'd been very heavy. I didn't want to purchase a new wardrobe when I was fat because that would have been a barrier to my losing weight," she reasons. So Bonnie imagined buying her first outfit as a reward for reaching goal weight. "It would be a very expensive, very sexy one-piece outfit for skiing and snowboarding," Bonnie muses, "and it would be red."

Bonnie practiced visualization just as she was going to sleep. This made her practice even more effective, because conscious defenses are down as sleep approaches, and thoughts are more readily accepted into the mind. This is really a hypnotic technique. Here's how Bonnie describes it: "I let certain images play through my mind just before falling asleep, or sometimes when I woke up during the night. The images had the quality of a dream, but were begun with a conscious wish. The first one was based on one of Lord Byron's poems, 'She Walks in Beauty, Like the Night,' which has been a favorite of mine since high school. I'd mentally let the words

120

of the first four lines of the poem float through my mind, and I'd think of myself as I wanted to be—at goal weight, walking freely and gracefully through a field with the moon shining down on the goldenrod.

"She walks in beauty, like the night
Of cloudless climes and starry skies,
And all that's best of dark and bright
Meet in her aspect and her eyes . . ."

"I wanted so much to be the person in the poem, and achieving my weight goal would be the first step. More than looking attractive, I wanted to gain an inner glow, and use that energy to help my husband and my daughters regain strength and enjoy life as much as possible after our tragic loss," Bonnie states.

Bonnie also used lots of positive visualizations about food, mentally planning exactly what she was going to eat for breakfast and how delicious it would taste. Occasionally, she'd actually create a new recipe and then make it for dinner the next day.

Focusing every day on being successful was the critical difference that helped Bonnie lose the last 15 pounds. "Visualization was a daily reminder of my goal. I was paying attention to what I wanted my life to be like as a KOPS member," she remarks. (Three of the visualizations that Bonnie used regularly are so effective that I've presented them below in the "Things to Do" section of Rankin's Reminders.)

Bonnie also made sure that her visualizations were supported by her actions. "A friend of mine was going through a divorce and was also dieting," Bonnie says. "She'd lost 50 pounds and had bought herself a new wardrobe. The problem was that she was miserable inside—she missed cooking and eating to the point that she gained back the 50 pounds and again wore her 'fat' clothes, which were still in her closet. I didn't know what to say to her except that I was extremely sorry. I knew what to do, though, and went home to totally reorganize my closet—I didn't want to have any 'fat' clothes to fall back on! I developed a whole new list of interests other than eating and food preparation by taking evening courses at a local college."

Bonnie's son, Martin, had always been health conscious, and he'd encouraged his parents to exercise and make good food choices. They'd ride bikes and ski together, and if Bonnie was in a weight-gain phase, Martin would try to motivate her to lose. So, it wasn't surprising that the first thought Bonnie had when she stepped on the scale the day she reached her goal weight was of her son. "I knew he was looking down on me and was proud of what I'd achieved," says Bonnie, choking back tears.

Two years have passed, and Bonnie has maintained her weight loss. Her husband took up skiing and has lost his excess weight, too. Bonnie is now the leader of a TOPS group and inspires her members. She teaches them the need to stay focused on their goals, and encourages them to visualize success every day and night.

A year ago, Bonnie was diagnosed with endometrial cancer. She endured the agony of the diagnosis, a battery of tests, and surgery before she could breathe a little easier. The good news is that the cancer hasn't spread, and throughout her ordeal, her TOPS pals were there for her. They sent cards, and their thoughts and prayers gave her the strength to stay on the program. Even though she wasn't allowed to exercise, she maintained her goal weight by eating sensibly. A month after surgery, she attended a chapter meeting wearing a new dress. Everyone cheered and shared her joy.

Bonnie knows that losing weight might have saved her life. "When I underwent the cancer surgery last summer, I was so thankful that I weighed 155. It would've been a much more dangerous surgery and a harder and longer recovery if I'd been 75 pounds heavier," she says.

Bonnie also used visualizations to help defeat the disease. "While fighting cancer, I imagined that all the tumors were successfully taken out of my body and that I was healing," Bonnie recalls. "As I was about to enter surgery, I imagined my husband and my two daughters standing very close to me, and all my friends—including the members of my TOPS chapter—were holding candles and standing in a circle around me. I felt safe."

Losing the weight has made life more precious than ever to Bonnie. For example, her son had two motorcycles that Bonnie and her husband now enjoy. "It was challenging to learn to ride, but now we often go to interesting places on them during the weekend. I probably wouldn't have done this at 230 pounds, but successfully losing weight has given me the confidence and courage to try new things," says Bonnie, a woman whose imagination, focus, and commitment has allowed her to overcome tragedy and live life to the fullest.

Rankin's Reminders: Visualization

- Whether they realize it or not, most successful people use visualizations to reach their goals. Some people daydream about success, which is a form of visualization. Others actually dream (in their sleep) about reaching goals. Rather then leaving this critical process to chance, however, seize control! Devise and practice visualizations to enhance power and achieve success.

- Visualization is a powerful training and motivational aid, used by many professionals. Bonnie is correct in pointing to one of the numerous pieces of research that show that visualization enhances skill learning. It was with this in mind that my colleagues and I at the University of London investigated whether visualization could improve temptation management for a group of alcoholics. This study, which was the central part of my Ph.D. thesis, showed that having alcoholics visualize resisting the temptation to consume an alcoholic drink improved their ability to actually do so in a real-life setting.

- Human beings are made to experience the world in images. It's true that a picture is worth a thousand words—seeing an image not only conveys information, it creates emotional and a sensory impressions. Moreover, the visual system is one of the oldest parts of the brain and predates the development of language and logic. Visualizations bypass conscious, logical defenses and penetrate deep into the psyche. This gives visual experiences, such as dreams and the imagination, tremendous power.

- Visualization not only enhances skill learning, it has motivational benefits, too. The image of *being* successful has hypnotic properties and advantages. If you can actually see yourself at a goal, then the mind accepts that this is a real possibility.

- When you imagine yourself doing something, you're actually practicing it physically. Many of the neural pathways involved in imagining resisting ice cream, for example, are the very ones used when actually doing so in real life. So imagining success is actually a method of reprogramming the mind and body.

- Words, thoughts, and especially images, carry emotions. Motivation is emotion, and experiencing motivating emotions each day is critical to success.

Visualization: Things to Do

1. When visualizing, try to find a quiet, softly lit spot. Relax, close your eyes, and imagine success. If you can't imagine success right away, persevere. Practice makes perfect.

2. You can probably easily visualize by simply closing your eyes and willing yourself to think of a scene. Sometimes this scene will be viewed as if through your own eyes, while other times an objective "outside-the-body" perspective will be taken. It doesn't matter which of these techniques you use, and you may even switch between the two.

   Likewise, you might visualize in full color, or maybe you'll see your mental images in black and white. Again, that's not terribly important, although the more vivid the visualization, the more powerful it's likely to be.

3. There are two types of visualization—skill enhancing and motivational. In skill-enhancing visualizations, imagine successfully completing an action. For example, imagine saying no to tempting foods, or making healthy choices at the buffet line, or exercising when you really don't want to. Motivational visualizations are more metaphorical and act like hypnotic messages. Metaphors are powerful because they bypass conscious defenses and go straight into the psyche.

   The first step in successfully using skill-enhancing visualizations is to compile a list of skills that you want to master. These might include the following:

- Successfully resisting temptation

- Practicing deep breathing when stressed

- Drinking water instead of soda

- Eating slower

- Serving smaller portions

The goal of these visualization exercises is to practice success, so focus on specifics. For example, if you're visualizing going for a walk, imagine putting on your workout clothes, walking out the door, and warming up; also, try to picture the scenes you'd see on the route. Always end by imagining the successful completion of the task, and feel good about your success.

Here are Bonnie's motivational visualizations. They're great examples of how to motivate and hypnotize yourself.

— **Climbing the mountain.** I'm walking through the foothills of a mountain. There are no trees, which means that I can see the top of the mountain—my goal. There are wildflowers blooming and the walking is easy (like losing the first 20 pounds).

The second stage of the climb is harder and steeper. There is mud, which causes me to slip. The dark trees obstruct the view of the summit (like losing the next 40 pounds).

The last stage of the climb is the steepest, but the light penetrates through the trees and I can see my goal. With renewed energy, I reach the bare granite surface of the mountaintop and realize that the view is worth all the effort of the climb (like losing the final 15 pounds and becoming a KOPS member).

— **Climbing the ladder.** I'm in a circus tent. It's dark except for the spotlight shining down on me. I steadily climb the ladder leading to the tightrope, rung by rung. Sometimes I slip, but I'm able to stop myself from falling, and I start to climb again. There are 75 rungs (pounds). I reach the platform, and then I'm ready for the next challenge—the tightrope.

— **The lifeboat.** My entire TOPS chapter is in a lifeboat. Everyone has an oar and the leader has the rudder. We're maneuvering between cold, angry waves and gargantuan icebergs made of lard toward a faraway beach where we see the faint glow of a lighthouse. Everyone must row if we're going to succeed.

4. Use Bonnie's metaphorical visualizations, or devise your own. Practice them daily, especially before going to sleep.

5. Discuss possible visualizations with others to get different ideas and feedback.

"Imagination is the beginning of creation. You imagine what you desire, you will what you imagine, and at last you create what you will."

— George Bernard Shaw, author

CHAPTER 17

✻

Countersabotage

What do you do when your spouse doesn't want you to lose weight, or your family members won't support a weight-control program? Claire Banaszak tells her story of how she dealt with these problems; along the way she provides marvelous insight into exactly who the *real* saboteur is.

● ●

"Don't Let Them Hook You: Claire Banaszak"
BY HOWARD J. RANKIN, PH.D.

At five feet tall and 180 pounds, Claire Banaszak had been a yo-yo dieter for most of her life. "I'd been on diets for years," says Claire. "They never worked."

Yet when Claire turned 62, about the same age that her parents were when they died, she got really scared—especially when she started to have health problems herself: She suffered from hypertension, and her cholesterol level was nearly 300. "Life is short, so with one foot in the grave and the other on a banana peel, it was now or never," she recalls.

Part of Claire's problem was that she'd never had much external support. Her husband was quite happy with her weight and wasn't very supportive of Claire's efforts. "I really tried to lose weight for more than 30 years," Claire maintains, "but most of that time I just kept on gaining, thanks to the enablers such as my husband and other dear friends and family members. When you're accepted as you are, no matter how fat, it can actually be a hindrance. You fail to improve because you already have approval from others."

Many husbands and wives discourage their spouses' weight-loss efforts. Sometimes this sabotage is very direct, such as giving them chocolates on a regular basis; putting the spouse in high-risk situations, such as all-you-can-eat buffets; or insisting that high-calorie foods be kept in the house. Other times the sabotage is more covert, such as when they make it quite clear that they're disinterested in any weight-loss efforts.

There are several reasons for such spousal sabotage. Some people may feel threatened by a partner's weight loss—or even fear losing their partner—since weight loss is often equated with increased attractiveness. It may also be the case that they recognize the need to adopt a healthier lifestyle, but don't want to feel pressured to do so. Above all, weight loss is transformation, and such personal change can—and does—alter the dynamics of a relationship.

It's tempting to blame enablers and saboteurs for weight-loss failure. They make it more difficult in many ways, eroding motivation and offering easy excuses. "When loved ones constantly tell you that they love you just the way you are, it takes a lot more willpower and determination to stick to a program," says Claire. "However, it's when you can't accept yourself that you really decide to do something about the weight."

Claire's turning point came when she went to a TOPS retreat. Removed form her usual domestic setting, she could finally see that her husband was sabotaging her. More than that, she could understand how the sabotage worked, and what she could do about it. "I realized that my many years of failure were partly a result of the lack of support I got on the home front," she asserts. "After all, if my husband accepted me just the way I was, where was my motivation to change? I really needed acceptance for the way I *wanted* to be. In the end, I had to seek motivation elsewhere. I went to the TOPS retreat, got myself a mentor who is also a great role model, and went on from there."

Claire returned from that retreat motivated and determined not to make her husband's resistance to her weight loss an excuse. Her TOPS buddies had to keep reminding her of the fact that the only power her husband had over her was the power she gave him.

The retreat also provided Claire with some practical tips for reaching her weight-loss goal. "Since I wanted to lose a large amount of weight, I established smaller realistic goals to keep me moving forward. I did it all one step at a time, and it wasn't easy," she says. "But that's the whole point—it wasn't easy then, and it isn't easy now. The difference now is that my mind is set, and I'm all the healthier for it. This doesn't mean that I never have an ice-cream cone or a piece of pizza, it just means I *seldom* do."

Eventually, Claire lost 60 pounds, and she discovered something very fundamental about sabotage: "I now see that the real problem was with me. All dieters want the support of those around them, and most of all, we want the support of those closest to us—our families. I didn't get the kind of motivation I needed by being reassured that my family loved me just the way I was, but blaming my husband and other enablers was nothing but an excuse to not lose weight," Claire acknowledges.

Claire is right. The simple fact is that we *give* saboteurs and enablers power over us. No one can sabotage our weight-loss efforts unless we let them. Saboteurs can make it much more difficult to stay focused on a weight-loss program because they erode motivation. Yet *difficult* isn't the same as *impossible*. It becomes all too easy to use enablers as an excuse to fail.

As Claire says, "I see many people at meetings who are just like I used to be. They have the acceptance of family and friends, just like I had, and they use that acceptance as an excuse for not losing weight, just like I did. So I tell them, 'It's only when you wake up and realize that you have to do it on your own that success is possible. You have to realize that the help you need has to come from within, and you can't let anyone or anything get in the way of a healthier you. There are some things that no one can help you with but yourself—the power within begins with you.'"

So what is life like for Claire now that she's been successful in reaching her weight-loss goal? "My husband and friends love me the same, but now they admit that I look a lot better and a lot healthier," says Claire. "My husband is still big on cookies, candy, and other sweets, but these things are very bad for me, so I leave them alone—and he doesn't try to push them on me anymore. The hardest part about giving up these goodies is that I still have to have them in the house. It's been long enough now that it doesn't bother me as much anymore, but it would *really* bother my husband if the sugary stuff wasn't around. I'd like to see him make better choices—and *I* sure set a good example—but in the end, he'll have to decide. He'll only change his habits when he wants to."

Claire and her husband have now negotiated a situation where they each respect the other's right to eat whatever they want and pursue their own habits. They can't change each other's behavior, so they've both adapted. "Now my husband says, 'I'm getting myself some ice cream,' whereas he used to automatically get some for *both* of us," Claire reports. "I've learned to say, 'None for me, thank you,' or, 'I had my mind set on an apple or an orange.' I try not to eat in the evenings, but when I do, I choose air-popped popcorn or a piece of fruit. Preparing food is sometimes difficult, because I have to remember that not everyone is on a diet with me. Still, I've learned a lot about cooking meals in a healthier manner. Nothing is deep-fried anymore, and I've been doing this so long that no one seems to notice!"

• •

Rankin's Reminders: Countersabotage

- Several years ago I was giving a seminar on the subject of sabotage. Part of that seminar involved having participants write down the name of all the people who sabotaged their weight-loss efforts. There were various categories of saboteur: controller, supervisor, naysayer, and enabler. When the exercise was being discussed, one woman raised her hand. "There's one person who fits in all of these categories," the woman announced. Everyone in the group turned toward her, interested to hear who that person could be. "It's me," she said.

- Saboteurs work by hooking your own anxieties and doubts, so take some time to resolve these issues. People can't have power over you unless you give it to them.

- Address saboteurs directly. Some people might not even realize that they're being counterproductive. When you talk to them directly, you'll quickly discover who is unwittingly sabotaging you, and who has a specific agenda.

- Stay positive, and don't even listen to negative comments. If you can't hear something positive, don't hear anything at all. Only listen to the people you trust—those who have no agenda other than helping you.

- Get angry at those who would have you fail, and use that anger to inspire your efforts. Whatever you do, don't use the anger to shoot yourself in the foot.

Countersabotage: Things to Do

1. Make a list of those who sabotage you and note how they do so.

2. Devise strategies for dealing with each and every one of those people. Such strategies might include talking to them directly, avoiding them, or getting angry with them.

3. Identify others who can reinforce your sabotage-fighting strategies, either through emotional support or direct action.

4. Review your own attitudes and behavior with others to ensure that you aren't self-sabotaging or making it easy for others to derail you.

5. Realize that the buck stops with you: Others can only make it difficult for you if you let them.

"People never improve unless they look to some standard or example higher or better than themselves."

— Tryon Edwards, editor

CHAPTER 18

❈

Emotional Eating

Emotional eating plagues many people—in fact, it's one of the biggest factors in weight gain. As this story shows, emotional eating can affect people at all points on the scale, and it can be devastating—emotionally as well as physically.

● ●

"Feel, Don't Eat"
BY DAWN LECY

My weight has gone up and down all my life. I've never been terribly obese, but I've lost the same 25 pounds or so at least seven times. My problem is that I'm an emotional eater, and I've never known what a healthy weight for me should be. I've always compared myself to other girls and women in magazines, on TV, and in everyday situations.

I grew up in a small town of 3,000 in southeastern Minnesota. In high school I was a chubby girl who never had a date. In college I lost weight, thanks in most part to climbing the four flights of stairs to my dorm several times a day.

When I graduated from college, I got a job as a Christian day-school teacher. I moved to an even smaller town where there wasn't a lot to do. There weren't many people my age around, and I was bored, so I'd eat. Thankfully, I joined a local aerobics class.

I met my husband soon after, and I managed to stay a healthy size until after our wedding. But then I had to be the good little farm wife and make big meals and bake lots of goodies. Of course I helped my husband eat it all, and I gained weight as a result. However, I went to a hospital-sponsored support group right after our first anniversary and was able to lose the weight.

Then we decided to start a family—and the yo-yo dieting really began! We had a healthy daughter, and it took me about a year to lose the extra 25 pounds I'd gained while I was pregnant. But I did it in time for my ten-year high school reunion in 1990. I was proud to go back and wow my classmates—I was no longer the chubby teen.

A year later we decided to add to our family—*Yay,* I thought, *I can eat again!* We had our second daughter in 1992, and I managed to lose weight a little more quickly after giving birth this time. But then I gained the most I ever have when I was pregnant with my son, who was born in 1996.

No matter what size I was, even at my lowest weight (118 pounds on my 5'7" frame), I never thought I was thin enough; in my mind I was always fat. One particular day when I was painting one of my daughters' rooms, it got to be too much. I was feeling overwhelmed with the responsibility of being the mother of three young children and having a craft business at home, and I was frustrated because I didn't seem to be doing anything well. My thoughts turned to my weight. I was sure that if I could just lose the extra pounds once and for all, I'd be June Cleaver and my life would be perfect. So, the next day I called my sister-in-law, who belonged to TOPS.

In January 1998, I joined a TOPS group in Marshall, Minnesota. When I'd gone to other weight-loss groups, I'd never had to set a goal weight. Everyone just seemed to be competing to see who could lose the most, the fastest. But since TOPS requires members to set a goal, I went to the doctor for a physical. I told her that I needed to determine my goal weight. What was her formula for figuring it out? She simply asked me,

"What do you *want* to weigh?" I gave her the number I'd always felt was acceptable, and that's what she put on the sheet to send to TOPS.

Looking back, I see that I wasn't really ready to lose weight at that time, and I used lots of excuses to justify quitting TOPS—it wasn't convenient, my kids were too little, and so on. In hindsight, I didn't need to lose as much weight as I thought I did. At any rate, I quit after about six months.

Then some family issues from the past came up that I couldn't deal with, and I turned to food for comfort. The stress of life got overwhelming again, and for the next couple of years, I was mostly in denial. Even though I kept having to buy larger clothes, I did nothing about my weight gain. I remember feeling so ashamed of how I looked that I didn't even attend my 20-year high school reunion.

My mother has battled her weight for her entire life, and now she's very obese. I felt so bad for her as I watched the quality of her life deteriorate, and I knew that I needed to make some changes for myself unless I wanted the same fate. When I started to grow out of my size-14 jeans, I decided that this was a sign to stop what I was doing and take control of my life.

At about this same time, my mother-in-law was very excited because she had joined a TOPS group and had reached her goal weight. I kept telling myself that I'd tried TOPS before and I didn't find it helpful. I thought, *I have a college degree, and if I really want to lose weight, I can do it on my own. I'll just eat less and exercise more—this isn't rocket science!* But as my jeans got tighter and my mother-in-law became more enthusiastic, I decided to give TOPS another try.

I went to a meeting, and all the members were very welcoming. However, the part that hit home the most for me was when the KOPS members said their pledge—there were so many of them! They were all different heights and ages and body types, and they all looked slim and healthy!

I joined the Granite Falls TOPS group that very night, weighing the most I'd ever weighed as a nonpregnant adult. I found a different physician, who measured my body fat and helped me determine what a healthy size for me should be. She discussed my lifestyle, health history, and stress level, and came up with a goal weight that would be achievable and maintainable.

From the TOPS group, I learned that it's okay to take time out for me. I'm really accountable only to myself, my Lord, and my loved ones. Taking time to exercise almost every day is my biggest stress reducer. It helps clear my head, and gets things in perspective.

Awhile ago, as I was flipping through a family photo album, I noticed something interesting about myself. I'd see a picture where I thought I looked pretty good, but then on the next page would be another picture where I was heavier. Then I started checking the dates of the photos, and I realized that the ones where I looked heavy had been taken after stressful or sad times in my life. When things were rough, I'd gain weight. When times were better and I was making a conscious effort to take care of myself, I was thinner. I started to recall many instances of overeating due to emotional issues.

The pattern stretched back as far as high school. I remember going out with friends and wanting to fit in with the popular kids, and, of course, wishing for a boyfriend. On more than one occasion I'd go home feeling disappointed, and I'd head straight to the freezer for some ice cream. I'd fill a cereal bowl and pour lots of chocolate syrup on top, eating every last lick by myself. Then I'd feel nauseated and angry with myself, and I'd vow to eat healthy the next day. But tomorrow never came for me—I just didn't care enough about myself to change.

I also remembered that in college, when I had my first real boyfriend, I lost a lot of weight quite rapidly. My roommate was concerned about me, and my mother was also very worried, because this was around the time that Karen Carpenter died from anorexia. Of course when my boyfriend broke up with me, I went back to overeating and self-loathing. I was sure that if I had been "better," he would have still wanted to be with me.

Looking back, I saw that I always wanted approval from everyone. I hated conflict and couldn't stand the thought that people might not like me—or worse still, might be angry with me. As a result, I developed the habit of being the peacemaker, and only saying what I thought people wanted to hear. Loneliness, frustration, and anxiety were emotions I didn't want to deal with, so I shoved them down with food. Anger was about the only emotion I felt without turning to food—when I was mad, I'd clean. So that emotion was a good one to have once in a while!

A couple of years ago, I was doing a job that I absolutely hated, but it involved family, so I felt obligated to stick with it. It was one of the roughest times I've been through. The stress was intense, and since I'm the type of person who doesn't like to start a conflict, I did a few different things to try to cope. First, I took a lot of it out on my husband, which was very unfair to him. Second, I wrote in a journal. That was very helpful for me. I could claim my feelings, write them down any way I chose, and then move on. I also did a lot of praying, and reading of self-help books. I found a couple of quotes that put my problems in perspective: "Feel the guilt . . . and do it anyway," and "You wouldn't worry about what other people thought about you if only you knew how little they did!"

Finally, I learned to say no. From there I was able to talk to my family members and get out of the job that distressed me, and I felt that a huge weight was lifted. I found out that my quitting wasn't really the big deal I'd imagined in my mind—in fact, my family was fine with it. I had overestimated their reactions. This lesson was really reinforced for me when I was asked to do some substitute teaching a short while later. The timing was very inconvenient, but I hesitated to refuse. I thought that if I *did* refuse, the school might be angry with me and never call me again. Still, I summoned all my courage and said no. I was stunned to find out that not only were they *not* angry with me, they asked me again the very next week.

Now I feel that I have a better handle on my emotions, and therefore, more control over my eating. My self-esteem and self-acceptance have soared now that I've found coping activities other than eating, and I know that the changes I've made on the inside have helped me accept myself on the outside. I'll never look like someone in a magazine or on TV, but I'm content.

I lost 25 pounds after joining TOPS, and I reached my goal in August of 2001—right before my 15th wedding anniversary. This made my husband very proud. I also turned 40 that same month, and it was great entering a new decade feeling good about myself. I'm finally happy to be right where I am.

Because I've never been able to maintain a healthy weight, I know that it's essential for me to continue to attend TOPS meetings to keep the pounds off. And even though I have that college degree, I still learn new things almost every time I go to a meeting.

Rankin's Reminders: Emotional Eating

- Dealing with uncomfortable emotions by eating creates three problems out of one. First, emotional eating does *nothing* to dispel or effectively deal with the underlying emotions, which consciously and subconsciously continue to influence behavior. Second, because these emotions are not dealt with, the issues that create them remain unaddressed, and the lack of effective action lowers self-esteem. Third, emotional eating creates weight problems, which in turn lower self-esteem further.

- Any behavior that seems to protect hurt feelings and soothe the mind will be done often and compulsively. Moreover, because emotional eating can be a painful experience, it's very often done in an automatic and dissociative way. (Dissociation refers to the mental process of removing attention from immediate reality.) Consequently, emotional eating is often not under conscious control. Obviously, this is a recipe for caloric disaster.

- In the story above, Dawn identifies a common problem—avoiding conflict for fear of rejection and anger. This has often been identified as the most common fear, and also the most damaging one. Wanting everyone to like you is completely unproductive, because in the end, you end up pleasing no one—least of all yourself.

- For some, anger seems incompatible with love. It's certainly true that the immediate feelings of anger are incompatible with loving feelings, but that's a far cry from saying that if someone is angry with you they no longer love you. Yet this simple logical error is at the heart of the desire to please, and it can be crippling.

- The desire to please can be all-consuming precisely because it's a defense against rejection. It often leads to attempts to control other people by appeasing them. I once had a client with this problem who was a tennis coach. I always try to find metaphors to which my clients can relate, and on this occasion,

I used a tennis analogy. I explained it this way: "Interacting with others is like a tennis game. In your case, you hit the ball over the net to the other person, and then run around to their side of the court to make sure they can hit it back to you," I said. "You can't play both sides of the court. Just stay on your side of the net and let the other people in your life decide for themselves how, when, and if to hit the ball back to you."

When Dawn was able to stay on her side of the metaphorical net, she found that people didn't get angry and immediately reject her when she voiced her true feelings. This discovery was liberating. I've seen many clients over the years who have made the same discovery, and the rise in self-esteem that follows their newfound ability to assert themselves has been meteoric.

• The emotions that most often triggered Dawn's emotional eating were frustration, anxiety, and loneliness. Boredom and spiritual emptiness are also common triggers for bingeing and excessive eating. All of these emotions tie in to the feelings of rejection and abandonment—two extremely powerful forces.

  The best way to counter any of these emotions is through meaningful contact with another human being. It's the lack of contact that fans the flames of isolation and rejection. So call a friend, visit a colleague, talk to a family member, or do some volunteer work—make contact with anyone who will respond positively to you. Hiding yourself away and stuffing yourself full of food in agonized privacy will only make the feelings of abandonment and rejection even worse.

• Anger is another emotion that can trigger emotional eating. Many people are horribly confused by anger. They've been trained to believe that being angry is sinful, and thus, they feel guilty about it. Many people also wrongly confuse anger with hate. Know that anger is a natural reaction that occurs based on the perception of unfair treatment, and it's an important part of assertion.

- The feelings of tension and energy that are created by anger can be scary. Those who are used to feeling in control of their emotions are sometimes scared that they'll lose control of themselves. This is such a stressful idea that they'd much rather lose control of something less threatening—such as their eating. Millions of calories have been consumed in the fire of rage.

- People also go to great lengths to avoid facing their anger. One of the most common rationalizations used is, "What's the point? The offending person isn't going to change anyway, so why bother?" This assumes that the point of expressing anger is to bring about change in another person. It isn't.

   The act of expressing anger is primarily designed to preserve physical and mental health. Releasing the tension that occurs when you feel upset is physically beneficial, because keeping the lid on such a strong emotion takes an incredible amount of energy. It can be so draining that there's virtually no energy left for anything else. That's why depression, which is primarily a lack of energy, is often considered anger turned inward.

   Validating and managing anger is a psychologically healthy act of self-expression. No matter how it's rationalized, avoiding anger is a cop-out. Whether you admit it consciously or not, you know it's a cop-out, and this has a devastating effect on self-esteem.

- Food is a poor alternative to feeling. Fat, sugar, and empty calories might numb you, but they don't solve your problems or take away your emotions. Feeding your feelings might temporarily help you forget them, but facing them will set you free.

Emotional Eating: Things to Do

1. The first step in handling anger is to validate and accept it.

2. The next step is to release the emotion in a harmless way. This involves getting it out: Discussing it with others, writing it

down, or even talking about it into a tape recorder are all good means of getting the feeling out.

3. When you're feeling emotional, move around. Even if you don't have time for a full walk or workout, get moving for at least a few minutes. It's a wonderful way to release tension. No matter how bad you feel before you exercise, I guarantee that you'll feel better once you've worked out for at least 20 minutes.

4. When you feel emotions rising, make a conscious effort to focus on your breath, as controlling your breathing can calm you down. Drinking a glass of water can also help.

5. Connect with a supportive person. Just talking will help the emotion pass and will restore perspective.

"People who fly into a rage always make a bad landing."

— Will Rogers, actor an humorist

CHAPTER 19

❈

Planning

Alan Gordon's story shows that organization and planning are a critical part of weight-loss success, and these behaviors can be easily learned. You simply have to plan, and you have to plan simply.

· ·

"Perfect Planning Prevents Poor Performance"
BY ALAN GORDON

I accept responsibility for the weight problems I've had throughout my life. However, there's no denying that my family environment provided the perfect setup for obesity. Both of my parents worked, so from the age of six, coming home from school was always a time for me to eat. I'd spend time at my grandparents' apartment until my mother came home, and there I was treated to a bowl of ice cream, a cupcake, and a candy bar—every afternoon. I always ate a very full dinner with dessert, and then, to finish off the day, I'd either get or sneak a snack just before bedtime—usually milk and cookies.

Could it be any worse? Well, my grandmother also gave me a quarter each day, which allowed me to buy lots of penny candy on the way home from school. (Today I cringe just thinking about it.) This went on, day in and day out, for many years.

I became a latchkey kid in the fourth grade, which meant that my afternoon snack got larger. With no one to monitor my food consumption, I ended up eating dinner and dessert twice each evening, plus a snack. In no time I was huge—a 150-pound third grader.

I stayed in the 50- to 75-pound overweight range until I graduated from high school. Then once I was in college, my waistline expanded more than my knowledge. I ate between each class and added huge volumes of food to my diet—many times my evening snack amounted to half of my calories for the entire day. I just seemed to eat constantly. I grew from 250 to 350 pounds in about two years. Although I had some minor successes at weight loss, I always seemed to rebound and add the usual 10 percent more within six months of each weight-loss attempt.

After getting my weight down to 225 pounds by exercising and eating the exact same 1,200-calorie menu every day for a year, I went back to school for my master's degree. I then proceeded to gain weight until I was in my third year of a Ph.D. program. My weight escalated to 440 pounds, and it became a major issue. I left the program, and luckily, I found a job within a few months. I also joined a fasting program, and again, I had short-term success.

At that time, I met my future wife. I remember warning her that I had once weighed more than 400 pounds and that I wasn't sure I could lose weight and keep it off. We started dating when I was 275 pounds, married when I was 330 pounds, and nearly divorced when I reached my all-time peak of 505 pounds.

It's strange, but embarrassing moments didn't seem to faze me and never led to lasting motivation. People would do all sorts of cruel things: laugh, talk behind my back, snort like a pig, and moo like a cow. Once, when I was going to start an exercise program at a pool, some people screamed, "Watch out for the beached whale!" Another time, I went for a jog and someone yelled out, "What's the point? You can't run far enough to work off that amount of fat." Yet another awkward moment was stepping on a cattle scale to find out that I weighed 440 pounds (most regular medical scales don't have the capacity to measure this much weight)—the maximum weight measurement tolerated by my Ph.D. committee.

Worse, the scale operator had to wash cattle feces off the platform before I could get on it.

Later, I was asked to leave the Ph.D. program I was enrolled in. Many people suspected that I wasn't losing weight fast enough, and the administration wanted me out of the program. In private, I was told that I was an embarrassment to the faculty and they didn't want me associated with their good name.

While my skills in my chosen field meant that I never was without a good job for long, my life was miserable. I had no energy, so I'd frequently fall asleep at work—at my desk or even during meetings. I didn't know it, but I had severe sleep apnea. Before I was successfully treated, I lost a great job because I kept dozing off. I'm sure that my condition was also an issue at my Ph.D. institution, and was part of the reason for my dismissal. I was finally diagnosed and treated for sleep apnea after getting my current job, but it still took a few years of struggling before my weight started to come off and stay off.

What did reaching rock bottom look like? It was very ugly. At one point when I was nearly 500 pounds, I played a game of tug-of-war with some friends, and I ended up hurting my back—causing an injury that slowly progressed until I was unable to stand or sit for more than a few minutes at a time. This meant that I had to read my mail by lying on the floor of my office. A co-worker once walked in on me when I was in this position and screamed because she thought I was dead. The severe back problem went on for more than a year, during which time I couldn't imagine walking more than a block without grabbing on to a wall or signpost for support.

I first joined TOPS in 1982, but I came and went several times. It was only when I combined several methods of weight loss that complemented each other that success came my way. I generated this momentum (what I call "big mo") by working closely with a nutritionist and attending my TOPS meetings regularly. My nutritionist kept me focused on my TOPS program, and my TOPS meetings would help me follow through with my nutritionist. The balance worked well. These steps, combined with a very monitored and dedicated plan of dieting and exercise, have yielded great results.

Now, on the day that I write this, I've just run a corporate 5K in our office park, which I completed in 25 minutes and 56 seconds—an 8:22-per-mile pace. The change in my life, from pain and suffering to joy, is almost indescribable.

Now my idea of fun is the challenge of riding my bike 50 miles or mountain climbing in Arizona. My dreams used to revolve around food, and now they center on activity and accomplishment. Since I first started writing about my challenges in a journal, my list of achievements has grown. In 2000, I set and reached a meaningful goal. My boss decided that her team would attend a session of Space Camp. I was excited and scared by the opportunity, because I still weighed 290 pounds. As I read the brochures explaining the program, I saw the height and weight requirements: The maximum weight for the Space Camp simulators is 260 pounds. I was 30 pounds away from that weight, and there were only nine weeks until the event.

I decided that I *was* going to ride those simulators, so I cut my calories from 2,500 to 1,800 and exercised twice a day—taking care to use cross-training techniques to avoid injury. On the day that I departed for Space Camp, I weighed 259.75 pounds. I'd reached my goal! I rode those simulators and participated in every event. I was thrilled. I know that I couldn't have lost the weight without intense planning and preparation.

In 2001, my longest run was eight miles, and I thought that was going to kill me. I laugh about it today, because now I consider eight miles a modest run. In 2002, I ran two half marathons (13.1 miles each), a 30K (18.6 miles), and I recently completed my first full marathon (26.2 miles).

Even though I've controlled many of my old habits and have maintained the majority of my weight loss, there are aspects of the old Alan deep inside. Significant stressors caused my weight to fluctuate up and down between 200 and 230 pounds for most of 2001 and 2002. So why haven't I followed my traditional pattern of spiking right back up toward 550 pounds (500 pounds, plus 10 percent)?

The difference is that now I'm planning and executing, and I'm still attending my TOPS support meetings. In the past, I'd let one or more of these behaviors slip away, and then I'd ride the weight-gain roller coaster. Now, even a bad day has me exercising and ordering my food without any sauce or oil. The old Alan would eat a cake or something like that. But because I've kept core elements in place, it's been easier to recover from the backsliding.

The kitchen staff at my office know me by name—my assistant will call down and say, "Can you make a lunch for Alan?" and they know exactly what I want (steamed vegetables and a broiled chicken breast). When I'm invited to a lunch meeting, most administrative assistants in my company know to order me a special meal—but I always check, just in case. When I travel to conferences or meetings offsite, I often call the meeting organizer and ask for a specific menu. It's not wise to leave it to chance or to just assume that a vegetarian meal or a diet plate will be healthy.

I've experienced very few instances where someone refused to accommodate my diet. If that ever happens, I know that I can either find a deli or eat the emergency food that I always bring to off-site meetings. I'm actually amazed by how easy it is to get help, and I'm usually eating better than most people around me: At banquets, my food is always freshly prepared, not sitting under a heat lamp for an hour.

My preparation for travel is meticulous. When traveling by plane, I bring my own meal rather than rely on what's available at the airport. I keep all kinds of healthy food in my suitcase, and immediately upon arriving in my destination city, I find the local grocery store. I then jog over to purchase water, fresh fruit, and yogurt. I keep these items in a cooler that I bring with me. Additionally, I always have the following foods in my briefcase when I'm out of the office:

- A 3-ounce package of StarKist tuna in a pouch
- A high-protein energy bar
- A 3-ounce package of turkey jerky
- Soy nuts, balsamic vinegar, and gum

These healthy snacks keep me from making poor food choices during the day, and, combined with some lettuce, many of the items make great salad toppings.

I also check hotel Websites to see if they offer workout facilities, or I go online to find nearby health clubs. I bring plenty of workout clothes, and even a jump rope just in case I'm too busy to get to the gym. These habits are now so well ingrained that I do them automatically, and I can't imagine *not* being so focused.

When I'm invited out to dinner, I go to the restaurant's Website and look up the offerings. If it's a fancy place, I'll call my nutritionist for advice and suggestions rather than risk making an impulsive, unhealthy choice. This allows me to try some fun dishes rather than just ordering plain broiled fish and steamed vegetables all the time. I've actually called my

147

nutritionist from the restaurant table to review the menu! This always generates conversation with my dinner companions, but I'd prefer that this be the talking point rather than the fact that I weigh more than 500 pounds.

People often assume that I'm a naturally organized, somewhat compulsive person, but I'm not. If anything, I tend to be a little unfocused in most aspects of my life. If I approached my career the way I approach my health, I'd probably be the director of my company by now. It's because I'm *not* that organized in life that I have to go out of my way to aggressively plan my eating and exercise routine. I can't rely on autopilot when it comes to my health—I realized a long time ago that for me, autopilot means morbid obesity. So each night before I go to bed, I take some time to examine my plan for the next day. I pack my briefcase with this plan in mind.

Because it isn't in my nature to be well organized, I first made it a commitment, and then I practiced it until it became a habit. Now I almost feel lost if I don't plan this aspect of my life.

• •

Rankin's Reminders: Planning

- You can't leave matters to chance. As I said at the beginning of this chapter, you simply have to plan, and you have to plan *simply*. This isn't difficult to do. Like everything else, it just requires the decision to act.

- More planning means more success. The more aspects of your daily routine that are planned, the less room there is for getting off track. Some people are natural organizers for whom planning is effortless, and they have a definite advantage over those who aren't as disciplined. But like most other behaviors, planning can become a habit if practiced, even if it isn't part of your personality.

- If you always plan, then you won't find yourself in a bad situation. Alan says, "I've never had to eat something because I had no other options—never!"

- If you always have a plan, others will know what they should do to make you feel comfortable. For example, Alan's company used to serve cookies at afternoon meetings, but now they offer cookies *and* fruit.

Planning: Things to Do

1. Have a weekly meeting with yourself to map out the upcoming week's exercise and meal schedules. Record your plans in an appointment book, and review goals from the previous week to see what worked and what didn't.

2. At your weekly meeting, anticipate any special situations that may arise in the next seven days and plan a strategy accordingly. For example, if you're planning to have guests, then schedule time to exercise when it won't interfere with other activities. That way, you won't make an excuse for not doing it.

3. Never cheat. Instead, plan to allow yourself some treats. Another one of Alan's strategies is to "always plan to eat the fresh-baked chocolate-chip cookies when I fly. That way, when I smell them on the plane, I don't have to fight the urge."

4. Keep your travel items, such as your jump rope and exercise clothes, easy to find—or leave them in your suitcase (even if that means you have to own two of each item).

5. Ask for help—you'll be amazed by how much some people are willing to do.

"It is a bad plan that admits of no modification."

— Publius Syrus, freed Roman slave

CHAPTER 20

❋

Self-Control

Can willpower be developed? Are there certain foods that must be avoided altogether? How important is self-discipline in weight loss? Jerry Boudreau provides some important insight in his story of weight-loss success.

• •

"Willpower, Walking, and Water: Jerry Boudreau"
BY HOWARD J. RANKIN, PH.D.

"It's all a head game," says Jerry Boudreau about the weight-loss process. And he should know: He spent years battling what began as a 30-pound bulge, a burden that with age and circumstance threatened to take him into morbid obesity.

Jerry worked hard for a utility company. The physical labor that the job required kept this country boy, who grew up on lots of dairy products and meats, within sight of his waistline. But Jerry also played hard: He loved going on cruises, and it wasn't uncommon for him to gain eight pounds on a single excursion.

When Jerry was promoted to a supervisory position at work, his job became less physical, so the weight began to creep on. Then a few years prior to his retirement, he opened an ice-cream parlor with his wife—and gained another 20 pounds. Jerry, who stands 5'11", weighed 249 pounds.

"It really showed," Jerry admits. "One day I looked in the mirror and was shocked at what I saw. My face was fat, I'd lost my neck, and I had a big belly. I thought, *Oh my God, I'm too young to look like this.*"

Jerry decided right then and there to lose the weight. "Get naked and really look in the mirror," he advises. "It's the best motivation there is."

In the past, Jerry had dieted a little. He'd lose a few pounds and then gain them back, never really making a permanent dent in his weight. When he joined TOPS, however, he found that the positive reinforcement and encouragement he got from other group members made a critical difference.

The first thing that Jerry did was cut back on the high-fat foods in his diet. He ate dessert two nights a week instead of every day, and bacon and fried-egg breakfasts became an occasional treat rather than a staple. Ice cream, which had been a real weakness, was eaten "half as much, half as often." Jerry also started walking two miles every day. This regimen helped him lose some weight, but he was obviously going to have to do more to reach and maintain his goal.

After considering what he really needed to do to finally get his weight under control, Jerry bought a cross-country ski machine, despite the fact that he'd never cross-country skiied in his life. He became very focused on working out, and sometimes he'd even put his grandson on his shoulders for added resistance when he used the machine. "I decided to combine my lifestyle change with quality time with my one-year-old grandson. He loved the thrill of being up high, and I conditioned my body and reinforced my goals. He's now 13 years old, and he still remembers the time we spent together when I exercised. It formed a bond between us that's priceless," says Jerry.

Yet the truth was that no matter how much Jerry exercised, if he didn't get his large appetite under control, the weight wasn't going to come off. A critical feature of Jerry's approach to changing his eating habits was his willingness to *face* tempting foods and difficult eating situations, rather than simply trying to avoid them. "I think it's important to eat the foods you like. Of course you have to do so in moderation," says Jerry. "But if you just try to avoid your favorite foods, then it's an admission that you can't manage them, and they still have some control over you. That's when you're in trouble, because if you do happen to eat them, you'll be convincing yourself that you have no restraint. I've developed a lot more self-control by confronting challenging situations," he says.

"It wasn't easy to institute these changes in my life," Jerry confesses. "It took conviction and willpower to make exercise and healthy eating part of my routine. Yet when I made that shift, I suddenly found a whole new world, and a happier person inside of me. I find that I no longer have to think about pushing myself to go for a walk. Now it's just the way I begin my day. My new lifestyle energizes me and fills me with a zest for living that flows into all other aspects of my life."

The approach of confronting tempting situations really paid off for Jerry. He lost 50 pounds in a year and became the TOPS Connecticut King. He has maintained that weight loss now for several years. "Losing the weight meant a lot to me. I'm as proud of that accomplishment as anything else, and I've achieved a lot," says Jerry.

Now a motivational speaker, Jerry stresses the need to develop self-control, as well as other good habits—especially exercise and drinking water. "It's the three W's," he says. "Willpower, Walking, and Water."

Jerry still loves to cruise. Now when he goes, however, he's vigilant about eating, takes a couple of exercise classes per day, and generally doesn't gain weight. "Having worked hard for more than 35 years, I'm at the point in my life where I'm able to enjoy many travel experiences. Naturally, it would be very easy to forget how important my lifestyle is during the numerous cruises my family and I take—all types of rich foods are paraded before us. The scent alone is enough to overcome many people. However, as tempting as these foods may be, the way I feel about who I am now and how I got here far overpowers their lure. I taste and I enjoy, but I no longer overindulge. I've found that food never tastes as good as it looks, and the feeling of instant gratification I used to get from overeating no longer appeals to me. My willpower has become a way of life," he explains.

Now that he's in maintenance, Jerry allows himself the luxury of easing up a little on the weekends, knowing he has the self-discipline to keep the portions and calories in check. He doesn't feel deprived, because he has developed the ability to savor just a taste, rather than a full portion.

"There's nothing better than knowing that I've overcome an obstacle. It makes me feel like a true success," says Jerry. "Now I allow the energy of my willpower to guide me and focus my life into a healthy pattern, and I know that the best of who I am is yet to be."

• •

Rankin's Reminders: Self-Control

• Jerry's story is close to my own heart. When I was working as a researcher and professor at the University of London's Addiction Research Unit, the main focus of my studies was temptation management. At the university, a series of studies showed that it was possible to teach all types of addicts how to develop self-control. The fundamental principle behind this technique is well articulated by Jerry in his story. He says this about food: "If you just try to avoid your favorite foods, then it's an admission that you can't manage them, and they still have some control over you."

  If you have that attitude, then you're in real danger—because as Jerry points out, "If you do happen to eat them, you'll be convincing yourself that you have no restraint." In the field of addiction, this phenomenon is called the *abstinence violation effect*. You try to avoid the substances that are problematic on the grounds that they control you—but because you have that mentality, once you start using these substances there's no stopping. Crossing the line means unlimited and uncontrolled use.

• Food is not the same as alcohol or cocaine—or is it? While it's true that you do have to eat to live, whereas you don't have to drink or snort cocaine, there's no one food that's necessary for life. You don't ever *have* to eat French fries, ice cream, chocolate, pizza, or doughnuts to survive.

• There really are some foods that are toxic for you, and they should be avoided altogether. In many ways, it's easier to make the decision to avoid specific toxic foods altogether than to eat them in moderation. As St. Augustine said, "To many, total abstinence is easier than perfect moderation." He was talking about sex, but the principle is the same. Once you've made the decision to eliminate certain foods, you no longer have to even consider them. So, identify your toxic foods and cross them off your list. These foods will take you away from your goals, make your life miserable, and they might even kill you.

On the other hand, deprivation is the mother of failure. It's one thing to realize that a certain food is toxic and dangerous, and to eliminate it from your diet, and it's another to feel completely deprived. Lifestyle change implies that you're changing to a way of life that's manageable, possible, and desirable—not confining yourself to the monastery (or nunnery) of bread, water, and constant exercise. So while you might identify a couple of foods that are simply too toxic to handle, there are other tempting favorites that you'll want to enjoy on occasion. But remember: To be able to eat these goodies requires a degree of self-control. Even though doughnuts may not kill you, you can't lose weight if you eat them every day, or even every other day.

- A myth has developed recently in the weight-loss world about willpower. That myth suggests that willpower is irrelevant to weight loss. Part of this myth comes from people who think that willpower is a static trait that you either have or don't have, like a birthmark. These critics are unaware of the scientific literature that shows quite categorically that self-control *can* be taught. It's certainly true that some people are naturally more disciplined than others, but that doesn't mean that willpower can't be acquired. Moreover, clinical studies—not to mention common sense—dictate that the ability to resist temptation *is* an important weight-loss skill.

  The fundamental principle of self-control training can be simply stated like this: *Every time you successfully resist temptation, you're developing self-control.* So, when temptation arises, don't panic. See it as a great opportunity to develop self-control. Know that with practice and the right attitude, temptation *can* be controlled—and be assured that it fades over time.

Self-Control: Things to Do

1. If you're going to confront temptation, then you need to be proactive and deal with it head-on. This means that rather than waiting for temptation to come calling, you go out and hunt it down. Before racing out the door to the nearest doughnut shop in the interest of personal growth, however, it's important to embrace the principle of *graded exposure.*

    Graded exposure means that you can't bite off more than you can chew, literally and metaphorically. Experience is the best teacher, especially if you learn by trial-and-success rather than trial-and-error. (Trial-and-success shows you what to do, whereas trial-and-error only shows you what *not* to do.)

    In order to experience success, exposure to temptation needs to occur on a graded basis. This means that your initial exposure to foods and situations needs to be manageable, not overwhelming. As your confidence develops and you learn what it feels like to exercise self-control, more difficult situations can be confronted.

    Start by identifying five situations of increasing temptation. For example, your list for tackling ice cream might look something like this:

    •   Spend a few seconds looking in the window of your favorite ice-cream shop.

    •   Go into the shop, and then immediately leave.

    •   Go in with friends and wait while they eat and you don't.

    •   Go to the shop, have just a small taste of ice cream, and then go home.

    •   Go in, order a single scoop, eat half, then throw the rest away and leave.

2. Use visualization. In my doctoral thesis, I presented evidence that by visualizing yourself resisting food, you can increase self-control. So before you even expose yourself to tempting situations, imagine yourself successfully resisting the food. Using the example of confronting ice-cream as outlined above, a typical visualization unfolds like this:

> *Imagine yourself outside of your favorite ice-cream shop. See yourself going into the shop and looking at all the different flavors of ice cream. You can almost taste them, and you really want to eat one of them. Pick one of the flavors and order a small cone. See the server scoop the ice cream and hand it to you. Feel the texture of the ice cream as you enjoy the first bite.*
>
> *Then think about your goals—specifically, your motivation for losing weight. Visualize buying smaller clothes, being more fit, or not having to take insulin anymore. Remember that the temporary taste of the ice cream isn't worth derailing your motivation.*
>
> *Imagine yourself saying no to the ice cream. Now see yourself throwing the ice cream into the trash. Feel good about exercising self-control.*

3. There are various ways of manipulating the difficulty of the preceding exposure exercises. The following variables can make confronting temptation easier or more difficult. After you master one level of difficulty, continue to challenge yourself by manipulating these factors.

- Vary the social context. Generally, it's easier to avoid certain temptations in a group, because the dynamics exert extra pressure to be successful. It takes more willpower to resist temptation when you're alone, because then you're only accountable to yourself.

- Vary your physical state. Begin by confronting foods when you're relaxed. Then increase the difficulty by confronting temptation when you're hungry, stressed, or tired. It's a lot harder to resist overeating under these circumstances than when you're calm and satisfied.

- Vary the intensity of the exposures. Choose situations and foods that differ in their level of temptation. Confronting the more tempting foods and situations will obviously make the exercises harder.

4. Record your progress. It's important to keep a journal of your reactions and successes. Each time an exposure is completed, write down what the situation was (for example, "I walked in and out of the ice-cream shop"), and the ease of resistance. The ease of resistance can be simply measured by using a scale of 1 to 10, where 1 means "Very easy to resist," and 10 means "Almost impossible to resist." As you master one exposure, move on to the next level of increased difficulty.

    Over the years, I've found that many people don't give themselves enough credit for their performance or their progress. They demean the task on the grounds that it couldn't have been that difficult if they were successful at it! One is reminded of the Groucho Marx line, "I don't care to belong to any club that will have me as a member." Give yourself credit and observe how it becomes easier to resist with practice. You truly are developing self-control.

5. The final exercise of self-control is throwing food away. I'm not suggesting this as a daily tactic, but as an exercise in which you develop the confidence to know that *you* control food, not the other way around.

    This technique is designed to break your emotional links with food. It may be difficult to throw your favorite food away, but until you can, it has control over you. Many successful weight losers report a shift in their attitude toward food after using this technique. Whereas once they lived for food, they now see food as merely a means to an end.

    People often balk at throwing food away on the grounds that there are starving children in Africa, Armenia, or some other place. This is an attitude left over from the Depression era, when food really was a precious commodity. The notion that you should eat because others are hungry is quite ludicrous—it's not as if there's a global stomach and your eating nourishes others. Famine in Africa is not alleviated one iota by you, me, or anyone else overeating—whether we're having a pizza or a healthy gourmet meal. If you really want to help starving people in the world, don't buy junk food, and send the money you save to a reputable famine-relief charity.

Of course, the starving-children talk has absolutely nothing to do with famine or marginalized people. It has everything to do with guilt. There are many good reasons to eat, but guilt isn't one of them.

If you approach the task of throwing away a favorite food with the right mental focus, you'll succeed. Remember, this is an exercise to demonstrate your capacity for self-control. You *can* develop willpower. Once you have done so, you'll be able to eat your favorite treats in moderation. If you can't manage this temptation, then it's likely that this is a toxic food for you, and you're better off avoiding it all together.

Also realize that exposure to temptation happens all the time, and it isn't new to you at all. These exercises are designed to help you face temptation with a more positive mind-set—one that makes you a proactive winner over food, not a passive victim of it.

"All self-discipline might be defined as teaching ourselves to do the unnatural."

— M. Scott Peck, M.D., psychiatrist and author of
The Road Less Traveled

Chapter 21

Assertiveness

A major theme of this book is that social pressure is a powerful force that can be used for good or evil. Resisting the social pressure to indulge in unhealthy behavior is difficult. As the following story shows, it requires courage and commitment.

"Just Say No"

BY KAREN TRIMPER

Since January 1996, I've lost 102 pounds. I've gone from a size 24 to a size 8, and I've transformed myself from depressed and unhappy to empowered and confident. I'm a completely different person. I totally changed my life, and it was easier than you'd think—once I committed myself to losing weight.

I'd tried to lose weight before, but I'd never succeeded. There are several reasons why I think my resolve finally held this time. First, I watched a show about heart-attack prevention, and I answered yes to all the "at-risk" questions—I was at the point where the slightest exertion left me gasping for breath, and that scared me. Second, I joined TOPS. Finally, I told myself: *I can lose this weight if I just take control of my habits.* I'd said this a thousand times before, but it had never sunk in. I don't know why it worked this time, except that I was ready to love myself and give myself the power to do what needed to be done. I was ready to get in shape to play baseball, hike, camp, and ski—all the things I couldn't do when I was carrying around an extra 100 pounds.

I started very slowly, and I didn't exercise right away. Instead, I just cut down on the number of fat calories I was consuming. I switched to low-fat and fat-free foods where possible, and I tried to keep all my meals at 30-percent fat or less. It takes a lot longer to grocery shop when you're reading all those labels, but it's well worth it. I started taking my lunch to work and gave up one high-fat food at a time. The first thing to go was butter, and I haven't had the real thing since!

I started using I Can't Believe It's Not Butter! spray, which has no calories and no fat. There are a few other good substitutes, too—Molly McButter being one of them. Next I gave up mayonnaise. The substitution technique really worked for me, so each week I gave up something high in fat and substituted a healthier alternative. I still ate whatever my husband cooked for dinner, but in smaller quantities and with a salad.

I was making progress with my initial efforts, but I knew I'd have to start exercising despite my many excuses to the contrary: I couldn't afford to join a gym, I didn't want to go for walks alone, I didn't have time to work out, and so on. Finally, I trashed all those excuses and started walking. That was the extent of my exercise routine at first. When the weather got too bad to walk outside, I started watching aerobic and toning videos at home, modifying my workouts as my endurance and strength increased. I was amazed by how wonderful I felt, and how the weight was steadily coming off.

Learning to be assertive was probably the biggest hurdle in my weight-loss quest, but I managed to overcome this challenge by using positive self-talk. At times I've been my own worst enemy, and I knew that before I could convince others that I was serious about change, I'd have to believe that I was worthy. So I practiced looking in the mirror seeing myself as I wanted to be—not just my appearance, but my outlook, too. My attitudes about everything changed during and after my weight-loss journey. I found that I could focus on a goal and shut out anything that distracted me. The knowledge that I could really do it this time was empowering, and my self-esteem rose sky-high.

My positive self-talk gave me the confidence to say no to other people—family, friends, and complete strangers—but I also had to learn to say no to myself. In the past, denying myself certain foods made me feel deprived, and ultimately that feeling sabotaged every diet I'd tried. This time I had to realize in my heart and in my head that refusing some food was good, and I should be proud of the ability to say no the to things I'd always said yes to before. When I changed my outlook in that way, it became a lot easier to assert myself.

Learning to refuse food doesn't sound like it should be that hard, but when people are insulted because I've turned down their freshly baked pie or a piece of their birthday cake, it makes it very difficult. How many times have we all heard, "Oh, come on—one piece isn't going to hurt"? Some folks have a very hard time taking no for an answer, and at that point I have to stop thinking about their feelings and start thinking about my health.

I think one of the things that really helped me refuse food is the fact that I was very outspoken about my plan to change my lifestyle. I discovered that if I was honest with people about why I was turning down their offers, they were totally supportive. When my friends and family members realized that this wasn't "just another diet," they were so helpful that they'd even say no *for* me!

I also discovered that it's not *what* you say, but *how* you say it. If I was appreciative but resolute, people were very understanding. However, if I gave the impression for one moment that part of me really wanted to indulge, then the pressure increased. I couldn't have resisted that pressure if I hadn't learned to be positive and confident about my motivation and my ability to retain control of my behavior, my program, and my life. Without the commitment and positive self-talk, I could easily have allowed the social pressure from others to be yet another excuse to fail.

Even after I reached my goal weight, I had to stay focused on my ability to resist temptation. Right after I was crowned New York State TOPS Queen, I was very full of myself. It was flattering to have people tell me how beautiful I looked and how much they wanted to follow in my footsteps. It made me feel a bit too invincible, and I almost stopped saying no. People were always remarking that I could eat whatever I wanted to. "Look at you" they'd say. "You can afford to indulge." I always responded to them (and myself) with, "No, I have to stick with my plan. It got me here, and it will keep me here." I realized right away that being assertive was one of the reasons I'd reached my goal, and I couldn't stop now.

Being assertive also applies to dealing with your own resistance. For example, when I first started exercising I'd argue with myself every morning about getting out of bed to work out. I'd start out by saying that I had to get up and exercise, and then I'd think, *No, I exercised yesterday and the day before. I ate sensibly yesterday and last night, so I can skip a day.* Yet I knew how easy it would be to break my new habit, so I managed to get up and do it. Now I've been working out daily for nearly four years. I still have to talk myself into it on some days, especially on *Buns of Steel* day.

I reached my goal weight on July 7, 1997, and I can't begin to describe the feeling I had that day. It was the most incredible thing to watch my body change so drastically, and I can't even begin to describe how much better I feel now that I'm healthy and in shape. I still watch my fat intake, and I exercise for an hour every morning before work. In the spring and summer, I walk or ride my bike every evening; and in the winter, I hike. I started working out with weights a couple months ago, and I love it.

If you're strong and you love yourself, then you can find the courage to assert yourself and lose that weight. It's fun to see people I've known for years walk right by without recognizing me—but it's not only the weight loss that makes me seem different. Now I'm self-confident and extremely happy, and I'm sure it shows in everything I do.

• •

Rankin's Reminders: Assertiveness

- Losing weight is hard enough without having constant temptation thrust in your face by other people. But it's going to happen, so you have to be able to assert yourself firmly and without guilt.

- Being assertive isn't about other people; it's about you. Karen hit the nail right on the head when she said that being assertive doesn't just apply to resisting temptations served up by others, it also applies to dealing with your own resistance. Saying no to others is also saying no to yourself. This is an exercise in self-discipline.

- Most people want approval from others—what lengths are *you* prepared to go to, and what costs are you prepared to pay for the privilege of being liked? Will you put your popularity before your health, your self-esteem, or your goals? The simple fact is that if people don't like you because you won't eat their dessert, then there's something wrong with *them,* not you.

- The more you practice saying no, the easier it becomes. Moreover, the more you say no, the more you're training others to expect you to be firm.

- Being assertive means keeping control of your weight-loss plan. Don't give control to others: They'll hijack your program.

Assertiveness: Things to Do

1. Show appreciation for tempting offers, but refuse politely. Remember: It's not *what* you say, but *how* you say it that counts.

2. If necessary, explain that you're on a program to improve your health, and it's very important to you.

3. Be strong, and don't be apologetic. If you hesitate or are ambivalent, people will turn up the heat and pressure you even more.

4. If you're struggling, focus on the negative consequences of acquiescing: Not only will you eat unwanted foods, but your self-esteem will suffer, too. Think about that the next time you're facing temptation.

5. If the folks you hang out with make sticking to your plan too difficult, then find other companions who are more supportive of your goals.

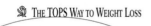

"It's impossible to fit in and stand out at the same time."

— Anonymous

🌹 🌹 🌹

✳

CHAPTER 22

Accountability

Accountability is a key element of successful weight loss and an essential part of what TOPS has to offer. Accountability doesn't just come to you, however. As the following story demonstrates, you have to seek it out.

· ·

"Someone to Answer To: Christi Smith"
BY HOWARD J. RANKIN, PH.D.

Although Christi Smith had been overweight ever since she was in the second grade, she never let her size stop her from having an active childhood. She loved to play sports—basketball, volleyball, and softball, to name but a few. She also enjoyed speed skating, and occasionally she skated with future Olympic champion Bonnie Blair. It's fair to say that Christi's weight never stopped her, it just slowed her down.

Christi followed in her dad's large footsteps. He weighed 350 pounds, and at the age of 45, it caught up with him. He died of a heart attack when Christi was just 14.

"My mother was the nursing supervisor the night my father died. She came home from work with my oldest brother and told me and my other brother that he was gone. I was obviously very upset—after all, I was Daddy's girl. The last words I spoke to him earlier that evening were 'I love you, Dad.' I miss him terribly to this day," says Christi.

Through her adult life, Christi's weight continued to climb, but she tried to maintain a positive attitude and not let it get in her way. "I'm a typical redhead—I'm stubborn," she insists.

Christi might have wanted to believe that her weight wasn't an obstacle to her goals, but that wasn't entirely accurate. Her dad had been in the military police, so in college Christi pursued a degree in law enforcement and had her mind set on a career in that field. She failed the physical agility test, however, so she abandoned her dream.

Christi was an emotional eater. "I used to have a very bad temper, and I'd get angry and eat," she admits. "Food provided me with comfort. Of course after eating to try to feel better, I actually ended up feeling worse, because it only made me fatter. So my self-esteem fell even lower."

During adulthood, Christi's weight climbed. She made a few short-lived attempts to lose the weight, but never made a lasting impression. She'd also fall into the perfectionist's trap. "Once I started overeating, I'd think, *What's the point of trying to lose weight? I'm so heavy already.* Then I'd feel guilty and ashamed, and I'd want more food," says Christi. "I'd be completely stuffed, but I'd continue to eat."

Considering her weight, which at this stage in her life was close to 300 pounds, Christi was lucky not to have any major health problems. However, she did have periodic migraine headaches, and she also experienced social pains. "I knew people were talking about my weight. Kids would laugh and mock me when I tried to walk. When I got on an airplane, I could see the other passengers thinking, *Please, God, don't let her sit next to me.* People would stare at me when I'd shop for groceries, as if they were judging what I had in my cart. I was often ignored by salespeople, because I guess they didn't think fat people had feelings. They'd serve someone who was thin before me, even though I was obviously there first," Christi recalls.

Christi's occupation made matters worse. She wasn't in law enforcement as she'd once hoped; instead, she was a baker for a large corporation, making cakes, doughnuts, and a variety of confections. "My job made weight-loss attempts even more difficult. It was easy to eat those goodies, especially when they were still warm out of the oven or fryer," says Christi.

The biggest stumbling block for Christi was that she wasn't too motivated to lose weight. She still had an active life, so it was easy to pretend that her weight wasn't holding her back. It was a combination of events, however, that changed her attitude.

When she turned 40, Christi realized that she was just five years younger than her father had been when he passed away. Since she'd followed in his medical footsteps as far as excess weight was concerned, she was genuinely worried that she might not survive past 45 either. "I knew that if I didn't get some weight off soon, I'd probably have a heart attack like my dad did. I'm very much like my father, and I was afraid of dying young. I couldn't do that to my mom," she says. "I also had a very good friend who had just died from a heart attack at the age of 38. So I knew it could happen to me."

Another turning point came when Christi was vacationing in Hawaii with her mother and a friend. They decided that they wanted to take a helicopter tour. "When we checked in, the woman asked us our weights. When I told her mine, she was very apologetic, but said I'd need to buy two seats. I was extremely embarrassed and wanted to cry, yet I didn't break down there because I knew it would upset my mom—I cried later, alone. In addition to the apology, the lady who waited on us had found a company who could accommodate me, but we'd already decided to do something else instead," says Christi. "This was the first time that I'd run into a restriction like this, and it made me think."

Christi decided to take charge of her weight problem, so she joined the local TOPS group. She also realized that she'd need some extra structure and initial supervision: "I knew that I had to be accountable—not just to the group, but to one particular person," she explains.

With that in mind, she approached fellow TOPS member Jewel Jones, a woman who had lost 140 pounds to reach her own goal weight. Christi knew that Jewel was a straight talker, and wouldn't mince words. So she agreed to keep a food journal and show it to Jewel each week.

"The second week, I showed Jewel my journal. On one of the days I'd eaten a bagel for breakfast. Jewel asked how big the bagel was, then admonished me and told me only to eat half next time," remembers Christi.

Each week Jewel would scrutinize Christi's journal and make very firm suggestions about how her diet could be improved. To her credit, Christi diligently recorded everything she ate. "There would be no point in not being absolutely honest. Jewel was trying to help me achieve my goals. If she was a little intimidating, that's what I needed. I took Jewel's comments very well," says Christi. "I'd never had this sort of accountability before, and it made all the difference."

Jewel helped Christi monitor herself for more than a year—and knowing that she was going to have to face Jewel was a huge deterrent for Christi. Early on in her program, she was still tempted by the doughnuts and pastries she was making during the night shift, but then she would think of Jewel and her other TOPS pals. "I imagined Jewel standing right there, watching me. It made it a lot easier to resist!" Christi laughs.

As time went on, however, Christi started to see the foods she was making in a different light. "I'd pull the doughnuts out of the fryer and be amazed at the rivers of grease flowing off them. Then I'd watch them getting dipped in huge mounds of sugar. I'd also see the frosting as one huge chunk of lard," says Christi. "Doughnuts didn't seem as tempting after that."

Within a year, Christi had lost nearly 100 pounds. Jewel had done such a good job that Christi was comfortable monitoring herself, having learned to choose healthier foods and proper portion sizes.

By this time, Christi had also been working out on a regular basis. In characteristic fashion, she sought the assistance of a TOPS member she admired. "When I knew I needed to do some form of exercise, I enlisted Marge Hough. She'd lost 91 pounds toward her goal, so I knew she could help me. I affectionately call her 'Sarge Marge' because she's very tough about making sure I exercise even when I don't walk with her," says Christi.

Within a few weeks of starting a walking program, Christi was covering at least four miles a day with Marge. When Marge suggested that the two of them walk a marathon together in October 2001, Christi reluctantly agreed. "I didn't really want to do the marathon that year, but before I knew it, I was training for it," she marvels.

Unfortunately, it was extremely hot on the day of the race, and Christi didn't hydrate herself properly. She suffered an asthma attack and severe dehydration, and she was taken to the hospital where she required fluids and oxygen. Undeterred, however, she was back the following year, and this time she finished the race with a blister as her only physical problem.

"Finishing the race felt great. I was so relieved to see the finish line! Next year I'm doing a triathlon, and TOPS member Karen Preston is going to help me train for that. She's the one who's encouraged me to do all of these crazy things. She's also very supportive and makes me feel good about myself and my ability to accomplish anything I set out to do. She's my major role model when it comes to fitness, and she's a real hero in my eyes," says Christi.

Christi has learned many lessons from her TOPS friends: Now she takes just one bite of the foods that used to control her, she exercises in response to stress instead of eating, and she understands portion control. Most of all, she's learned self-discipline through the efforts of Jewel Jones, Marge Hough, and other TOPS members.

"Self-discipline is very important to fitness and losing weight," Christi shares. "Nobody can do it for you. Other people can give you support, but you're the one who has to make the right choices to eat nutritious foods and exercise. It feels great to know that I have control over food now, but I wouldn't have been able to do it if I hadn't asked for help."

Rankin's Reminders: Accountability

- It's often said that keeping a journal is the key to successful weight loss. I disagree. It's not the self-monitoring that's crucial, it's the accountability.

  Frankly, most adults don't like the idea of being accountable. This is a function of a society that focuses on individual freedoms. We like to imagine that we operate on our own and don't need the intrusion of other people's opinions. Even though *accountability* may be a dirty word and a concept that we don't like, it's essential when trying to change behavior.

  If you're going to be egotistical about weight loss, you'll probably fail. Humility may be a disappearing trait in contemporary society, but that doesn't mean it's not vital for success.

- There's a limit to how accountable you can be to yourself. In truth, self-monitoring is useful in observing patterns of behavior, but unless you share your observations with someone else, there's no accountability value.

- In the story above, Christi seeks out accountability. One of the features of this story is that it highlights the necessity of asking for help. Christi was active in identifying appropriate people who were willing and able to be her mentors, and she took full advantage of their willingness and their advice.

- Being accountable to an individual, rather than a group, has merit. Personal relationships increase accountability—provided you're answering to a person you respect. If you find someone to act in this capacity, the motivational value increases. (This is the reasoning behind the sponsorship concept in Alcoholics Anonymous.)

Accountability: Things to Do

1. Keep a food and exercise journal. Write down as much information you can about what you're eating, when you're eating it, and how you're feeling. Keep track of frequency and intensity of exercise.

2. Identify a mentor. He or she should be someone you respect who will speak honestly to you. You might need different mentors for eating and exercise like Christi did. If you can't find a mentor, then the group will have to suffice.

3. Visualize your mentor's response when you feel tempted to deviate from your goals.

4. Offer to be a mentor to others. This role reversal will help your own efforts.

5. Practice accountability in other areas of life.

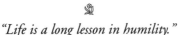

"Life is a long lesson in humility."

— James M. Barrie, playwright and novelist

CHAPTER 23

✳

Goal Setting

Goals are the map with which to find success. This story shows how setting small, incremental goals can lead to big payoffs.

• •

"The Next Step: Jim Draeger"
BY HOWARD J. RANKIN, PH.D.

When Jim Draeger had a garage sale, he decided to let his Levi's go. He hung his many pairs of blue jeans in different sizes on a rack in his driveway—a testimony to his gradual weight gain. Now he couldn't find jeans in any department store that fit him.

Not that Jim was overweight as a child. On the contrary, he was really skinny back then. Over the years, however—especially after the age of 35—the weight started to creep on. His girth started to grow by about 6 pounds a year, which meant that by the time Jim was 45, he was up more than 70 pounds. This put a total of 250 pounds on his six-foot frame. "I accepted the weight gain as a normal part of aging," Jim explains. "I didn't think there was anything I could do about it."

Jim resigned himself to the idea that he was powerless over the weight that was physically draining him and deflating his self-esteem. There was nothing he could do about the weight that made him potbellied, and sometimes the butt of jokes. So he laughed about it. Laughter deflected the subject and allowed him to control the criticism.

As Jim kept on laughing, he kept on expanding, too. When a bunion forced him to have a foot operation, however, the presurgical screening produced a nasty surprise. A physical showed him to be on the verge of adult-onset diabetes, and his doctor suggested that once he had completed his six-week post-op recovery, he should come back to discuss diabetes medication. Jim was terrified, and he knew that he had to try to lose some weight.

"My stepfather, whom I greatly admired, died of complications from diabetes. He, too, was overweight, but he was also very stubborn," Jim says. "Despite being a very intelligent man, he simply didn't want to accept the fact that he needed to lose weight. He was very childish and defensive about it, and it did him in."

Jim had the operation and was sent home on a heavy schedule of painkillers. While sedated he realized the effects of his abusive lifestyle. "I saw, with a clarity that I'd never previously experienced, what was preventing me from leading a fuller life," remembers Jim. "I had visions of the heavy ale I'd been drinking, and the bowls of ice cream and piles of pizzas I'd consumed." For the first time in his life, Jim accepted responsibility for his weight gain, and realized that *undoing* it would be his responsibility as well.

The first thing Jim did was to learn about diabetes by reading books and getting as much information as possible. Then he set his first goal: *No weight gain during the six weeks of postoperative recovery.* He was very concerned that the six-week recovery period would derail his newfound motivation, since he was going to be immobile and bored—a good recipe for added girth. So he used his recovery period to plan his weight-loss strategy.

Goal setting has always been important for Jim. As a tile contractor, his work follows a logical progression, so he's used to thinking of reaching goals in sequence. He used the same strategy in his weight-loss efforts.

Jim realized that he'd have to wrestle the task of food preparation away from his wife, a gourmet cook and pharmacist who didn't think that her husband was really committed to losing weight. He found the solution to this problem through a company that provided home delivery of premium frozen foods. Jim had been ordering from this service for some time, but only from the back of the catalog—which featured many desserts high in calories. When he looked through the front of the catalog for the first time, he found that the service also delivered healthy, low-fat foods. Moreover, the catalog also listed diabetic-nutrition information for each meal, making it easier for Jim to make wise choices.

For the first few weeks, Jim relied on the catalog's healthy products. He also set the following goals:

- Reduce calories to 1,600–1,800 per day.

- Switch from daily beer to red wine twice a week.

- Eliminate ice cream and pizza.

- Do some resistance exercises three or more times a week.

Jim says, "I tried to set specific goals that were within reach. I'd set many small goals that would lead up to a larger project being completed. Achieving results with smaller goals encouraged me to continue with my weight-loss program. It wasn't as rigorous as it might sound. I did enough of the right things, enough of the time, to maintain good results."

Within the first three weeks, Jim lost five pounds, despite his immobility. Encouraged by this success, he couldn't wait to start exercising. Walking, however, was a problem: He still couldn't make it around the block. Jim did have an old 12-speed bike, and he thought that riding it might help get his exercise program in gear.

Prior to his operation, Jim had driven to a local park to ride. When he got there, he found that he could barely reach the handlebars, and he couldn't make it over the first knoll without having to get off the bike. He was shocked to discover what poor shape he was in. After his operation, he was more determined than ever to get back on his bike. So within three weeks of his surgery, Jim was riding his bike in that nearby park. It didn't take long before he was riding as much as 90 minutes a day on paved trails.

Several pounds later, Jim joined his local TOPS group, encouraged by his mother who was a long-time member. He lost six pounds in each of the first two weeks. By the time he went back to the doctor to discuss his diabetes, he'd lost 20 pounds and significantly reduced his blood-sugar level. At his next checkup, no medication was needed, and six months later, Jim's blood sugar was completely normal. By that time, he'd lost more than 70 pounds.

It was his bike riding that offered the most challenging opportunity. As with other areas of his program, Jim set incremental goals for his performance. After he'd lost more weight and could actually ride a short while around a the park without getting exhausted, Jim set the following goals:

- Within a week, ride around the lake without getting off the bike.

- Within the month, ride over steep hills without getting off the bike.

- Within another week, ride over those hills in a higher gear.

"These were hurdles that I set for myself," Jim says. "Accomplishing them gave me a mental payoff. As I achieve more, I set higher goals for myself."

After losing the weight, Jim bought a mountain bike as a reward for his efforts and spent all summer riding at the park. He was able to get higher and higher up the hilly terrain. "The higher up you get, the skinnier the people get," he muses.

In the winter, Jim bought a new high-end bike for street riding. He enjoyed the camaraderie and support of fellow cyclists, and eventually joined the Santa Rosa Cycling Club. "The people in the club are focused on maintaining good health in order to pursue their passion for riding," he maintains. "I find it easier to pursue my goals in a group of like-minded people. They're continually challenging themselves, and I find this inspiring."

Jim lost more than 70 pounds in all, reduced his blood sugar, and effectively managed his propensity to diabetes. He did that by focusing on short-term goals and setting mental challenges each week. Some of the permanent changes he made were:

- no longer eating lunch out;

- only taking one trip through buffet lines at restaurants;

- eating fish for dinner four to five times a week;

- buying a half-gallon of ice cream no more than once a month;

- restricting his intake of cheese and other dairy products;

- never drinking sodas (Jim looks at sodas as being about as good for you as cigarettes!);

- eliminating fast food;

- rarely drinking beer; and

- eating one plate of food for dinner, not two or three.

Jim has also derived motivation from unusual sources. He finds what might be best described as "reverse inspiration" from observing people who are failing at weight control. As Jim says, "They remind me of how important it is to stay focused and how glad I am for my success. It's easy to get complacent, which is why I keep attending TOPS meetings."

Jim also finds inspiration in the fast-food industry. He's angry with these companies for what he sees as corporate greed at the expense of customers' health and the well-being of the nation. This anger makes it easy for him to avoid fast food. After all, if you're angry enough, you can give up anything.

Jim rides a lot now, including 100-mile treks, a feat that was unimaginable when he was overweight. In fact, one of Jim's current goals is to ride across the United States as part of a cycling group. Such dreams are now within Jim's reach. He has truly reached the top of the mountain, and he did it one step at a time—by setting small, manageable goals.

Rankin's Reminders: Goal Setting

- Goals are guidance mechanisms that help direct everyday behavior. So it follows that what you're doing today should be related to what you want to achieve tomorrow. Yet too often, there's little connection between today's actions and tomorrow's aspirations.

- Short-term goals are stepping-stones to long-term goals. The short-term ones are more important because they drive today's behavior. Without getting it right today, we can't realize our dreams tomorrow.

- Goals should be realistic, feasible, and manageable, and they should be written down. Setting goals that can't be attained is pointless.

- Goals should be incremental, and they're most effective when they can be expressed as objective behaviors. Keep breaking goals down into smaller and smaller units until you derive ones that can be achieved. For example, if you set a goal of walking three miles, five times a week, and you're unable to achieve that, then change the goal to something smaller that can be achieved—perhaps two miles, three times a week.

- Goals aren't set in concrete. Review yours every week, and build on your successes—don't lament failure.

- It's better to be successful at small goals than unsuccessful at large ones.

Goal Setting: Things to Do

1. Write down food, exercise, and other health goals. These should be expressed as specific behaviors. For example, write: "Reduce total cholesterol to less than 190, and walk for 30 minutes, five times a week."

2. Break each behavioral goal down into small steps.

3. Know what your goals are at any one time, and focus on what needs to be achieved each day.

4. If you're having difficulty reaching a goal, try to break it down into smaller ones until you find a level you're comfortable with.

5. Find appropriate people with whom to share goals. They will provide motivation, accountability, and feedback.

"This one step—choosing a goal and sticking to it—changes everything."

— Scott Reed, author

Chapter 24

Journaling

When I visited Owensboro, Kentucky, for the TOPS state meeting in the spring of 2002, I met Anola Sinnott for the second time. I'd met her a couple of years earlier and had thrown down a challenge that she really took to heart.

"The Write Stuff: Anola Sinnott"

by Howard J. Rankin, Ph.D.

Anola Sinnott had a difficult childhood, taking the brunt of her mother's physical and emotional abuse. Unfortunately for Anola, nobody knew at the time that her mother had a brain tumor that created her unpredictable, aggressive behavior.

Anola learned to deal with her mom's anger by escaping into books. She'd read anything available . . . but she'd also *eat* anything available. By sneaking and hiding food, Anola felt that she had some control over a part of her life. As a result of this pattern, Anola was overweight during her school years. She was also tall, so she really stood out.

Anola had no friends, and self-esteem that was below sea level. For one thing, she was embarrassed to take anyone home. For another, she didn't think she could be a good friend. After all, she didn't believe she could be good at *anything*. And it didn't help that her grandmother was an anorexic woman who pounded her emotionally about her weight. "I received a barrage of messages that I was useless. I was so low I'd have had to look up to see a snake," Anola recalls.

Anola took her first part-time job at the local five-and-dime store. When she graduated from high school, she took a secretarial course and then landed a clerical position at a hospital, where she's worked for the last 27 years.

Just before her 21st birthday, Anola finally escaped her abusive home and married Mike. At that point, she weighed 218 pounds. Mike had a son from a previous marriage, and in the early stages of the relationship there were the typical conflicts that occur in a blended family. This didn't help Anola's emotional eating, nor did the fact that she and Mike had completely different schedules. Her weight began to climb, and by the time their daughter, Brittney, was born, Anola weighed 257 pounds.

Things weren't destined to get much easier. Mike and Anola had just bought their second house together when Mike began to suffer from severe rheumatoid arthritis. He went from being a vibrant man who ran five times a week in order to maintain a 100-pound weight loss, to a completely disabled one. So Anola became the breadwinner while Mike stayed home with the kids. Anola was working 60 hours a week with little time to exercise or focus on healthy eating.

Working, eating, and sleeping seemed to be all that Anola did for the next several years. When she was stressed, she'd revert back to sneaking and hiding food—the same pattern she'd followed as a child. Her bingeing became all too frequent, and when she was feeling especially upset, she could eat her way through two pizzas. On a few occasions, her husband opened the refrigerator only to find that the ingredients he'd bought for dinner had already disappeared. This was rare, however, because most of Anola's bingeing occurred outside the home. To everyone around her, it seemed that she hardly ate anything.

"My husband was never judgmental. He was always accepting and never made me feel the way my mother did," says Anola. However, Mike also increased his eating and eventually regained all of the 100 pounds he'd previously lost—and then some.

In 1996, Anola was diagnosed with sleep apnea. She'd already fallen asleep at the wheel several times, but she'd been fortunate enough to slide gently off the road rather than ram into a tree or a telephone pole. Her blood pressure was "almost at stroke level, even on medication," and she weighed 390 pounds.

When Anola's insurance changed, she was required to get a physical from a new doctor. When the results of her blood tests came back, the physician called Anola back to his office for a stern lecture. "He told me that if I carried on the way I was going, I wouldn't live to see my grand-children grow up. I wouldn't make it past 50; and even if I did, I'd be a full-blown diabetic," she confesses. "He told me to decide what I wanted— to live or to die.

"I left in tears, went home, and immediately hit the refrigerator. Then I realized that this was stupid—I had to stop. I'd heard everything that doc-tor had told me from other people for the past 20 years. He just wasn't very nice about it, and I guess that's what it took," Anola concedes.

"During this period, I was very depressed. I felt as if I couldn't do any-thing right, and I even gave up my faith. I was so ashamed that I didn't think I deserved to be loved by anyone—even God. Besides, I couldn't stay awake at church, and I couldn't fit in the pews," says Anola. "I thought the only thing that I'd ever done right was marry Mike and have a daughter. Yet I didn't even believe that I was a good mother because I was always working and never home."

I didn't know Anola's story when I first met her in her hometown of Louisville during a TOPS International Recognition Day. She had been a TOPS member for several years, renewing her membership each year, but only going to a few meetings before she'd quit. By chance she attended a seminar in which I suggested the value of writing thoughts and feelings— as well as food intake and exercise—in a journal.

"A therapist had once told me to write a letter to my mother, outlin-ing what I'd liked and disliked about my upbringing," Anola shares. "I'd written it but never sent it. My younger sister read it and was stunned, because she'd never realized how much abuse I'd taken from my mother. As the oldest, I'd run interference so that I'd get the lion's share of the mis-treatment, instead of her. Still, writing the letter to my mother didn't really help me a whole lot, so when I heard the talk about journaling, I was doubt-ful that it would work for me."

After the seminar, Anola told me just that. So I asked her to make her journal more personal. "I still had my reservations, but then I immediately went to lunch and made a healthy choice—a salad rather than the buffet. I went back to my room and started my new journal," recalls Anola. "I wrote, 'Dr. Rankin, this won't work.'"

For the next two weeks, Anola wrote faithfully in her journal. She always started it, "Dear Dr. Rankin," and she always expressed the same idea—"this won't work." Eventually, however, she started to write about different things, such as how her day had been and how she was feeling. Soon she was carrying her journal everywhere she went, recording her thoughts and emotions throughout the day.

"Once I got into a routine, I was writing *everything* down, especially all my feelings. I would yell and scream to you, Dr. Rankin," Anola says. "Sometimes I might write four lines, sometimes I'd write 15 pages. I unloaded everything and went deeply into a number of issues."

After a while, writing in her journal became a substitute for eating, and venting emotions on paper became a healthy release. Anola also started writing prayers in the journal—she'd rediscovered her faith and her self-esteem. "When I felt really bad, writing helped me get the emotion off my chest and always made me feel better," she says. "Sometimes I was very formal, sometimes I was less so. Sometimes I had to think about what I wanted to say, and other times it just flowed—I couldn't write fast enough. No matter what, I always felt as if I were writing to my best friend. I don't think it would have worked as well if I'd simply written 'Dear Diary.'"

Anola wrote in her journal all but one day in the 18 months after my challenge to her. She regularly reviewed what she'd written, and reading her journal helped her understand her thoughts and emotions. During those months, Anola lost nearly 100 pounds.

Anola's husband, Mike, also shed 80 pounds during the same period. One reason for their success is that they both kept separate food diaries, an effective technique as long as they showed them to other TOPS members. "We needed to share the food diaries at TOPS meetings, otherwise we simply wouldn't write down any poor choices, or we'd ignore them," Anola explains.

Today Anola is the leader of her TOPS chapter. Although her diaries contain very personal details, Anola has read some of them to other members.

This has inspired some of these people to start their own journals. Theirs begin: "Dear Anola."

"My journal has been my savior," Anola asserts. "Not only have I used it to control my eating and express my emotions, it's helped me understand much more about the relationship between my thoughts, feelings, and actions. It has also restored my self-esteem. Dr. Rankin, you've become one of my best friends, even though you might not know it!"

. . . .

Rankin's Reminders: Journaling

One of the wonderful privileges of being a professional speaker and therapist is that occasionally people take what you say to heart and turn a chance comment into a life-changing challenge. Much of the time, speakers and even therapists don't get any acknowledgment that their suggestions have been helpful. So when I get feedback—like I did from Anola on that day in Owensboro—it's really rewarding and magical.

- There's real value in journaling. Writing down your emotions not only releases them from your mind and body, it makes them tangible. After all, unexpressed feelings are ill-defined feelings. Writing about your emotions gives them shape and meaning, making them easier to manage.

- One of the major themes in this book is the critical role of other people in all meaningful aspects of change. I find it very interesting that Anola couldn't just write in her journal, she had to address a real person—me. When she writes in her journal, she's having a conversation with me, even though I'm a thousand miles away and completely unaware of what she's writing. That conversational style allows her journal to become like a confidante that's always available and attentive, and a repository for her most difficult emotions.

- Anola and her husband also kept a food diary, which is a completely different type of journal. Food diaries are most useful when they're shown to other people, as highlighted in Christi Smith's story (Chapter 22).

Journaling: Things to Do

1. You don't need to buy a fancy book to record your innermost thoughts. You certainly can if you want to, but Anola used 99-cent yellow notepads.

2. Make it a habit to write every day. It doesn't matter if you only jot down one sentence—just write something.

3. Address your diary to someone. You don't ever have to show it to that person—Anola has never shown her journal to me. Please feel free to write yours to me if you so wish.

4. Review your journal entries at least once a month. Your reactions to the entries of the past make good entries for today. Notice patterns in your thoughts, emotions, and behavior.

5. Keep your journal handy throughout the day to write down thoughts as they come to you. Thoughts and feelings fade and might be forgotten or minimized if left until later. If you can't take your journal with you, make notes on bits of paper and transfer them to your journal later on.

"I am carrying out my plan, so long formulated,
of keeping a journal. What I most keenly
wish is not to forget that I am writing for myself
alone. Thus I shall always tell the truth,
I hope, and thus I shall improve myself."

— Eugène Delacroix, artist

CHAPTER 25

❋

Food Control

Losing weight requires controlling food intake. Unfortunately, managing food doesn't happen automatically—you have to work at it. Tory Magnusson describes the process in the following story.

. . . .

"Eating to Live: Tory Magnusson"
BY HOWARD J. RANKIN, PH.D.

When Tory Magnusson was a freshman in college, she returned home for Thanksgiving. As she got up from the table to get a second helping of mashed potatoes, her father, who'd never made a comment about her weight before, said, "Tory, you need to watch what you eat. You're getting a little heavy."

Tory was devastated. "I went upstairs—in tears," she says. "I could hear my parents arguing about his comment. My mom said, 'She knows that she's gained weight, and she doesn't feel very good about herself to begin with. Don't make it worse.' But my dad said, 'Well, a girl her age shouldn't be getting that heavy. It's not healthy.'"

Tory didn't realize that others thought of her as "heavy." That was in part due to the fact that she'd never really been overweight. All the way through high school, Tory had been very active in sports, so her weight had always been within reasonable limits. But when she went off to college, her eating quickly got out of control, and the pounds started piling on fast.

"I'd grown up in a town of 600 people," Tory explains. "The nearest restaurants were 45 minutes away. Then I moved to a big city that seemed to have a million places to eat. I was a poor college kid, but I always had enough money for pizza."

Tory gained 25 pounds during her freshman year. Although she lost the weight over the summer, when she returned to college, the bad eating habits came back, too. Within a month of starting her fall semester, she could no longer fit into the new blue jeans she'd worked all summer to conquer.

It was during that same year that she had a life-changing experience. One evening she was in her dorm room, studying biology. "I heard this voice in my head," said Tory, "It was telling me to call home."

So Tory dialed her parents, but there was no answer. A few minutes later, the same inner voice encouraged her to call again. On the eighth ring, her dad answered. "Why did you take so long to pick up the phone?" Tory asked.

"We've just finished harvesting beets, and I'm very tired. I was in bed," her father replied.

Tory usually talked to her mother when she called home, but Mom was out. So Tory and her dad had an unusually long phone conversation that evening. At the end of the call, her dad said something that he had never said before: "I'm very proud of all that you've done—at school, at your job, at everything." At the end of the call, he said, "I love you." He didn't say these words often, and they gave Tory a good but strange feeling,

Tory went back to her studying. Three hours later, a tearful resident advisor came knocking at her door. Tory somehow knew what she was going to say: "It's my dad, isn't it?" she asked rhetorically. "He's passed away, hasn't he?" She was right—her dad had died of a heart attack.

"The Lord knew that I needed to speak to him," Tory says today about that fateful evening.

Over the next three years, Tory gained more than 60 pounds. One time, at a regular checkup, her physician was very blunt with her: "You're going to have the same heart attack that killed your father," she said.

"I was very hurt," Tory recalls. "It was the wrong time to tell me such a thing because I was still so devastated by my father's death. It was about the worst thing she could have said to me, and it actually discouraged me. I just wanted people to love me."

Tory found reassurance from her fiancé, who loved her unconditionally. When she was married, Tory weighed 230 pounds. A year later she weighed almost 250.

By this time, Tory was the activity director of a retirement community. She was very lively during the day, but at night her body ached. "My feet hurt so bad that I wanted to cut them off. I also had shoulder and neck pain. Occasionally, I'd literally have to crawl to the bathroom because I had no energy," she says.

The residents of the community made comments about her weight. She overheard one person say, "For Tory's size, she sure can move." When she arranged a fashion show and her mother was one of the models, another resident remarked, "I bet you wish you looked like your mother!"

All of these comments hurt. Although Tory always had an air of confidence, her self-esteem was fragile. She felt resigned to be overweight forever because the task of losing weight seemed so overwhelming.

"One day I flipped through some photos of myself. I looked really old. Here I was, four years out of high school, and I looked like I was 40," Tory recollects. "I was eating horribly, and I was drinking a couple of 20-ounce Mountain Dews a day. I hated all my clothes, and I hurt. I knew I couldn't do it on my own, so I asked God for some help. I asked Him to give me a tool so I could lose the weight."

Shortly thereafter a resident in the retirement community asked Tory whether there was a local TOPS group. Tory had never heard of TOPS, so the resident suggested forming a group, and asked if Tory would be interested in joining.

By the fall of 2000, Tory was a member of the TOPS group started in the retirement center. "I'd always looked at the big picture before, and I'd get discouraged. A couple of weeks into TOPS, I realized that I didn't put this weight on in a couple of months, so I didn't need to try to lose it that fast," she says.

Tory had lost a few pounds when her husband suggested that they both join a fitness club. By January, she was working out three days a week on her way home from work. She says, "The first time I tried the step-aerobics class, I turned beet red and thought I was going to die. I was so slow compared to the others. I left in tears and vowed that I'd never go back." Tory returned again the next day, however. Her strategy was to adopt a positive, cheerful demeanor that sometimes fooled even her.

At her highest weight, Tory thought she could still do a cartwheel, and she launched herself toward the ground with both hands outstretched. "I couldn't get my legs up in the air, and I almost broke my wrist," Tory admits. Once she lost 60 pounds, she tried again—this time with success.

Giving up soda, drinking ten glasses of water daily, restricting eating out to just once a week, and exercising all established weight-loss momentum. But what really made a huge difference was a mental tactic: "I changed my thinking," Tory says. "I decided that I had to be in control of food—not the other way around. I started to do everything I could to reinforce the notion that I was in charge." With this in mind, she did the following:

- In restaurants, she'd immediately have the server box up half of her entrée.

- She drank two to three glasses of water with every meal.

- She didn't eat past seven o'clock in the evening.

- She never had second helpings.

- She avoided high-calorie and fatty foods.

- She left the dining area as soon as she was finished with a meal.

The new rules Tory set for herself were strictly observed. She planted a saying: "There's no food worth being fat for," firmly in her head, and she reminded herself of this every time she had a craving or headed to the kitchen out of boredom.

"I never felt starved," Tory notes. "In fact, I realized how little food I really needed."

Tory lost 90 pounds in ten months and has now dropped 110 pounds in all. "When I weighed 248, I wasn't playful anymore. I was scared. But now I'm full of energy, and I know my boundaries with eating," she states. "I feel good knowing that I can be in control. Food doesn't call me anymore—I go to it when *I* choose."

There's something else Tory does. Call it repayment or call it faith, but it's something she does religiously. "I pray for a release from temptation, and I thank God for the gift of getting my health on track again," Tory says. "Then I ask Him to help me have one more day of control."

* *

Rankin's Reminders: Food Control

- It's important to eat to live, rather than the other way around. That's not to say that food can't be enjoyed, but it should certainly be managed.

- You can't lose weight if food controls you, so focus on staying in control of your food intake. See it as a battle that must be won, and be aware of the consequences of letting food be in control: excess weight, low self-esteem, and less energy, to name a few.

- Realize that the positive effect of food is fleeting. The pleasure in food is the taste, which typically lasts a few seconds. Any pleasure from the *effect* of food is dangerous, because it implies that food is being used as a drug to achieve a certain feeling. Under these circumstances, food can become addictive.

- Develop rules for maintaining control. Focus on the speed at which you eat, be more patient, and watch portion size.

- Start small—you can always get more. You aren't going to starve.

Food Control: Things to Do

1. Eat slower, and start with smaller portions. You can always go back for more if you're truly hungry.

2. After a main course, wait 20 minutes before eating anything more. It takes that amount of time to feel the effects of eating, during which time hundreds more calories might be consumed.

3. Drink water as the first response to the temptation to indulge.

4. Don't eat after 7 P.M. Resolve fades as the evening wears on.

5. Practice these skills in a group. When you do so, they reinforce each other.

"Bad men live that they may eat and drink,
whereas good men eat and drink that they may live."

— Socrates, philosopher

🌹 🌹 🌹

CHAPTER 26

❋

The Magic of Exercise

I couldn't write this book without at least one story specifically focused on exercise. Lisa's account of her journey to fitness is typical, and it highlights some important aspects of exercise that shouldn't be overlooked.

• •

"Energized: Lisa Lee Jones-Garner"
BY HOWARD J. RANKIN, PH.D.

Lisa Jones was very active as a child. She played a variety of sports, loved to dance, and had a black belt in karate by the age of 14. However, even though she was raised in Oregon, her family had southern roots, and dietary preferences to match.

Lisa developed poor eating habits. She often wouldn't eat at all and would have to be bribed to eat by family members. Her grandmother, who was raised during the Depression and went hungry many times, actually paid her five dollars per barbecued Kentucky Fried Chicken leg she ate. Grandma also encouraged Lisa to drink all the fresh milk she could, claiming that these foods would make Lisa "big and strong," not bony and unhealthy like she was. So when Lisa did eat, she chose predominantly dairy products, especially chocolate milk, which eventually became her nutritional nemesis.

When Lisa was 17, she stopped all her physical activities—dancing, karate, marching band, and softball. She was going to college and wanted to dedicate all of her time to her studies. Her weight gain in the first year of college was not the typical "freshman 15," but an alarming freshman 80. She'd stopped exercising, yet she continued eating as if she were working out three hours a day, six days a week.

During her college years, Lisa's weight fluctuated between 240 and 280 pounds. When she tried to lose the weight, she was often successful for a short period, typically losing about 30 pounds before regaining it all, but the problem was that any weight-loss progress she made didn't stand a chance against what she describes as her "chocolate-milk fetish"—she'd frequently drink four quarts in a single day. By the time she graduated from law school, she was 5'7" and weighed 279 pounds.

After graduating, Lisa found herself managing the office of a rheumatologist. She herself had suffered from rheumatoid arthritis from an early age, and she wasn't feeling very good now, either: "I felt tired, depressed, and old," she says. "I felt like I was about 91, not 31."

One of the clinic's older clients told Lisa of the difficulties she was going through, and laughingly told Lisa not to get old because it was no fun. When Lisa told her that she already felt old and revealed her age, the client was taken aback. Lisa agreed that most of her problems were due to her weight. The client then mentioned the local TOPS group, and introduced her to a chapter member, Becky Sander.

In the fall of 1998, Lisa joined TOPS, although somewhat ambivalently. "Part of the reason for my slow start was that I still wasn't convinced that I could lose weight," she says. "I told myself that I would attend to support my mother, who is very obese and nearly homebound because of her weight. She only goes out of the house for TOPS meetings and doctors' appointments. It took a while to get to know people, but once I did, I looked forward to going. I started to believe that I really could lose weight, too. That's when I started putting everyone's great advice to work."

Lisa is a dog lover, and about the time she was joining TOPS, a fellow dog lover, Faye, suggested that Lisa join her on a hike with their dogs. Faye had seen Lisa at dog shows, and she assumed that she was in reasonable shape. What she didn't know was that after those shows, Lisa would go home and drop from exhaustion. When Lisa apprehensively asked about how difficult the hike was, Faye replied that it was "easy."

Lisa agreed to do the hike, but it turned out to be anything but easy. It was seven and a half miles, much of it uphill. She struggled mightily. "The beginning of the trail, before crossing the river to go up the mountain, is one mile, and I was asking if we were there yet before we'd even reached the river! When I asked how much farther, Faye just kept on walking and said, 'Not even close.'

"I plodded along very slowly, and I was well behind Faye the entire hike," Lisa continues. "Most of the time, I couldn't see her ahead of me. I was breathing so hard that I could barely talk. Her German shepherd, Sheba, would come back periodically to check on me, and I kept thinking, *Yep, Sheba's worried I'm going to drop dead from a heart attack.* I became convinced that she was one of those animals that can sense illness and disaster, and from the look in her eyes, I was a goner!

"My fat little dog, Mr. Scotty, was giving out, too. His tongue was hanging out like a cartoon dog, and he was barely waddling. After five miles, when we were about to begin the two-and-a-half-mile descent down the mountain, my hips were freezing up and I didn't think I could take another step. I felt extremely fatigued and my legs were giving out. I reached a point where I simply couldn't move. It was getting dark, and I started to panic. I thought I was going to die on that mountain. I finally made it down, although by then it was pitch dark and freezing. A hike that should have taken less than three hours had taken me nearly five."

The experience frightened Lisa. "I was depressed. I couldn't believe I was that weak. After all, I'd always prided myself on being active and strong. I fought boys instead of girls at karate tournaments—girls were always underestimated, and I thought it was amusing to win against the boys. I was proud of the fact that I could make it through a three-hour karate workout and barely break a sweat. What had happened over the years that suddenly I couldn't walk a few miles? I knew I was fat, but I'd always thought I was still strong. It was a wake-up call that I was seriously out of shape," she admits.

In the spring of the following year, once again Faye asked Lisa to go on a hike. "I told her that I couldn't walk seven miles, and I didn't want to go with her," says Lisa. "She said that we'd take a short walk around the neighborhood, so I agreed, secretly thinking that I could survive this time because there'd be phones, houses, and fast food nearby!"

Faye lied, however, about the "short" part of it, and at her pace there wasn't time for phones or fast food. "The walk took two and a half hours, and I estimate it was about six miles. I was getting shin splints from walking on the pavement, and I got blisters on the bottom of all my toes because I was wearing garden clogs!" Lisa remembers. "The next time Faye wanted to walk, I objected and reminded her of the previous two occasions I'd walked with her, and the catalog of injuries I'd sustained."

But Faye said that this time they'd walk around the golf course, a loop of about 2.2 miles. They were joined by another friend, who was one of Faye's regular walking companions.

"I made it around once and was behind both of them the entire time," Lisa remembers. "About every quarter of a mile, they'd stop and call back to make sure I was still alive. I made it, but I decided to stop after one loop."

Yet within six weeks, Lisa could walk around the course three times— more than six miles. Within two months, she was up to four laps—close to nine miles.

"I played a game to see how many times I could complete the circle," Lisa shares. "When I became accustomed to walking, I did this course a minimum of four times every day. A few times I actually did six rounds— about 13 miles!"

Lisa had become self-conscious about her appearance, and she avoided being seen, if at all possible. "I'd always take the back streets and use the rear entrances of buildings so I wouldn't be noticed," she says. "I avoided people at all costs."

In addition to her shyness and social phobia, Lisa was also depressed. The fatigue and lack of energy that characterize depression only made Lisa eat more. And of course, the more she ate, the more depressed she became. "When I'm depressed, I don't care how I look. I just want to do the only thing that gives me pleasure—eat," Lisa confesses.

For these reasons, Lisa and Faye didn't walk every day—they walked every night. They'd often start walking around 10 P.M., and they'd go for more than two hours. Their commitment to their nightly ritual was almost unshakable. There were a couple of times when Lisa simply didn't want to go, turned the light off, and hid under the covers, pretending to be asleep. On those occasions, her mother would rouse her out of bed to walk.

Faye and Lisa walked at a brisk pace. Lisa's dog, Mr. Scotty, would make the first lap, and then he'd scurry under her truck and whine until he was let into the cab. When they did another lap and passed the car again, Lisa could see Mr. Scotty laid out, fast asleep with his paws in the air.

The walks meant much more to Lisa than simple calorie burning. "Exercise made me happy and cheerful. It completely changed my mood and gave me energy," Lisa declares. "I felt like a kid at the end of each walk, and I had a real endorphin rush. In fact, Faye and I would often end the evening by playing at the nearby playground. We'd play on the swings or stretch our muscles on the monkey bars, and once we made ourselves so dizzy on the merry-go-round that we had to sit for a good 30 minutes before we could go back to the car. When I finished my workout, I had so much energy that when I got home it would take me an hour or so of doing chores to unwind."

This extra energy and boost in mood were critical to Lisa's weight-control efforts. She'd been raised to think that food was necessary to feel good, and she'd eat anything to elevate her spirits. "The effects of my exercise were mainly to give me energy and improve my mood to the point where I could easily manage my food. I had no cravings and much more control. Today, the mindless eating is gone," she says. "Mood adjustment is the reason I walk, more than calorie burning. I feel so energetic afterward. People notice a difference in my personality, too. I'm more tolerant, positive, and surprisingly physically active after exercise. After being depressed for so long and at times feeling so fatigued that I couldn't even comb my hair, the energy surge I have after exercising is like finding a miracle cure."

From the spring of 1999 until that fall, Lisa lost 72 pounds with her nocturnal walking. In November of that year, Lisa took a full-time job and had to cut back on her walking. By January, 2000, she was walking "only" three miles per day. By the end of that year, she had lost another 20 pounds—reaching her goal of a 100-pound total loss.

Exercise also helps Lisa manage her perfectionism. Occasionally, if she violates her stated goals for the day, she overeats. "I have a tendency to think, *I've blown it for today, so it doesn't matter,*" she says. "Then I have a big gain. So if I find myself heading down that path, I simply allow myself the few extra bites and figure them into the calories for the day. I don't obsess about it; I walk. When I don't exercise, I don't have the energy, and I'm much more at risk of not being able to keep it under control. And I always ask myself, *Is this food worth it? Do I want to walk an extra two miles to eat it?*"

. . . .

Rankin's Reminders: The Magic of Exercise

- Exercise is obviously a key component to weight control and health in general. It bestows many benefits apart from the burning of calories, and in the myopic quest for weight loss, these are sometimes forgotten or ignored.

- If there was a pill that provided as many physical- and mental-health benefits as exercise, people would be fighting over it. As if reducing disease risk and morbidity aren't enough, exercise increases metabolism, stamina, endurance, and quality of life. It also elevates energy levels and mood, which is the main point of Lisa's story.

- It's difficult to overestimate the effects of exercise. When energy is low, defenses are down, willpower is reduced, and the body seeks more energy through extra calories—a recipe for a major problem. The simple act of taking a walk can keep such problems at bay.

- Exercise can also offset natural energy slumps that occur in every 24-hour cycle. These slumps generally happen in the middle of the afternoon and late in the evening. The evening slump is best dealt with by going to bed. Walking for a short while can offset the afternoon slump and save hundreds of calories.

- By increasing energy and mood, exercise also increases self-esteem. Because self-esteem is raised by *doing,* exercise is psychologically beneficial.

- Lisa's story highlights, yet again, the value of other people in facilitating weight-loss efforts. Peer involvement may be especially crucial with exercise. In the above story, Faye certainly pushed Lisa—sometimes too hard. But Lisa will admit that without that encouragement, she wouldn't be where she is today—happier and almost 100 pounds lighter.

The Magic of Exercise: Things to Do

1. Keep a daily record of energy and mood levels.

2. Observe patterns in the relationship between energy and mood.

3. Observe and record the impact of exercise. What happens on the days when you work out? How do you feel during the following 24 hours? How does that compare with how you feel on the days you don't exercise? Do you manage food better when you have more energy and are in a better mood?

4. Exercise can offset natural energy slumps. If at all possible, take a short walk when you feel yourself fading—especially in the afternoon, which is a high-risk time for the consumption of unnecessary calories.

5. Find workout buddies who can challenge you and help develop your exercise program.

"As I see it, every day you do one of two things: build health or produce disease in yourself."

— Adelle Davis, author

CHAPTER 27

❋

The President's Story

When LaNeida Herrick got married, she wasn't overweight. Her husband, Henry, was in the Navy for the first three years of their marriage, and when he left the service, they moved out of the suburbs and onto a farm. There the Herricks had easy access to dairy products and LaNeida's favorite food of all—whipped cream.

"LaNeida Herrick"
BY HOWARD J. RANKIN, PH.D.

"We really hadn't had much opportunity for whipped cream when I was a child, so once I got to the farm I was in heaven. I actually baked pies just to have something to put it on," LaNeida jokes.

It didn't take long for LaNeida's weight to escalate. The farm lifestyle, along with her five pregnancies, didn't help her waistline. Before she knew it, the quintessential caregiving farmwife, mother, and Sunday-school teacher was up to 300 pounds.

"I was always giving to everyone else, but I wasn't doing anything for myself," LaNeida says. "I realized that this had to change."

LaNeida answered an advertisement for TOPS in the local newspaper. "When I got to the meeting, they told me that too many people had answered the ad, so I couldn't join. They asked me to come back the next week," she recalls. "I'd made such an effort to get to the group, and I knew that if I left without joining, I'd never come back. So I told them in no uncertain terms, 'I'm not leaving.'" LaNeida's persistence paid off. Despite initial reluctance from the group leader, she convinced them to sign her up.

LaNeida's determination and persistence were an asset to her weight-loss efforts. Even though she weighed more than anyone in the group when she signed up, she became the chapter queen that year, beating out the second heaviest member by less than a pound. Yet TOPS did a lot more for LaNeida than help her lose weight. As it has with thousands of others over the years, it helped restore her self-esteem.

Capitalizing on her enthusiasm, persistence, organizational drive, and charisma, LaNeida became a very successful area captain and then a coordinator. "Helping others and developing the organization meant a lot to me," she maintains. However, throwing herself into her TOPS duties deflected some of the energy that should have been directed toward her own weight-control program, and before long the pounds were coming back—and fast.

A turning point in her struggle came when she attended the first-ever TOPS retreat in the state of Washington. At that time, Imogene Welch was the only retreat director. "I learned a lot at that retreat. First, I realized that I was feeling pretty sorry for myself because I was an only child whose parents had died young, and life had been hard for me. Second, I realized that I didn't have to lose weight for anyone but me—that was quite a revelation. Finally, I saw that in all the time I'd spent helping others, I had lost myself," LaNeida says. "I found myself at that retreat."

A short time later, LaNeida met a lady named Mary Wallace who had lost 100 pounds with TOPS. Mary proved to be an emotional support and an inspiration, and she gave LaNeida some practical advice, too. "Mary adopted me. She told me that if I lost 20 pounds a year, I could lose a 100 pounds in five years," she recounts. "When I was concerned about taking so long to lose weight, she wisely advised me that it was better to lose slowly and keep it off, than lose quickly and put it all back on again." Thus advised, LaNeida did indeed lose 100 pounds in five years. She has maintained that loss for 25 years, and Mary has remained a lifelong friend.

As she climbed within the organization, LaNeida spent more and more time away at meetings and conventions. One benefit of this was that her husband spent more time with his kids than he might have been able to otherwise. LaNeida's husband and five sons have always been supportive of her, regardless of her weight.

One time, LaNeida got a call from her son Mitch's teacher, who told that another boy had taunted Mitch. "The teacher told me that the kid said, 'Your mom's fat!' and my son replied, 'That's just the way we like her,'" LaNeida says with a smile.

As LaNeida's enthusiasm and skill became recognized within the TOPS organization, she acquired more responsibilities. She became regional director of the Washington, Oregon, Iowa, Idaho, Alaska, Montana, and California chapters, and she was elected to the board of directors in 1992.

"TOPS has certainly changed my life. I've traveled to places I never would have seen otherwise, I've met thousands of wonderful people, and I'm comfortable addressing an entire convention, whereas before I couldn't have spoken to ten people in a room," she declares. Of course she has also helped hundreds of people reach their weight-loss goals, and she's played a key role in the development of the organization to which she has given so much.

LaNeida eventually became good friends with TOPS founder Esther Manz; after that, she became very close to Betty Domenoe, who followed Mrs. Manz as the second TOPS president. In 2002, LaNeida was elected president—she's only the third person to hold this office in TOPS history.

LaNeida still goes to weekly meetings at the same chapter that almost lost her on her very first visit 40 years ago. She has maintained her infectious enthusiasm and total dedication to the TOPS concept and organization, which she leads into the new millennium with characteristic drive and compassion.

"We make a living by what we get, we make a life by what we give."

— Sir Winston Churchill

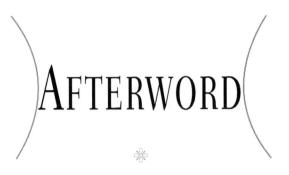

AFTERWORD

✳

It's my hope that you've been inspired and informed by reading this book. It's also my hope that you've learned that we're all "works in progress," and that striving for physical improvement entails psychological and spiritual growth. No one is exempt from this challenge, and as soon as you think you no longer need to focus on health and enlightenment, life will conspire, in one way or another, to give you a rude awakening. Each of us needs to commit to continue the quest of self-discovery. That's a requirement of all of us—even health experts, psychologists, and authors of self-help books.

I want to share a little about my weight-loss story and my recent travels on the journey down the path of self-discovery. In terms of pounds lost or medical struggles, my story isn't very dramatic, and it doesn't compare with some of the other accounts in this book. But I *can* you tell you how I've evolved to become the best I can be.

The two women in my early life, my mother and older sister, were my introduction to weight concerns. Neither was overweight, they just thought they were. This was an era when women not only *wanted* to look like fashion models, they thought they *should* (unfortunately, times haven't changed very much). In our house, matters weren't helped by the fact that Twiggy, the aptly named anorexic-looking British supermodel and actress, actually attended the same school as my sister. There are billions of women in the world and maybe 20 of them are supermodels—and even *their* photos are computer enhanced. Ladies, I'm sorry, but the odds are against you.

As an athletic boy blessed with a lean body type, I never had to think about my weight. I knew about how much I weighed, but it never occurred to me that my size was, or ever would be, a problem. Up to my college years, I was active in sports and ate whatever I wanted.

As both an undergraduate at the University of Nottingham and then a postgraduate at the University of London, I became less active and enjoyed the standard college fare: beer, peanuts, fish and chips, and chocolate, not necessarily in that order. That is until one day, when I looked in the mirror closely for the first time, and I saw that, yes, indeed, I was overweight. Not just overweight, but fat—there was an extra layer circumventing my middle! This was a huge shock. I was an athletic lad who excelled at football (soccer in the U.S.), rugby, and cricket, and I simply had never thought of myself as anything other than the epitome of athleticism. Yet here I was, 30 pounds overweight.

I was thus thrown back to my main source of reference about dieting (and in those days it was definitely *dieting,* not *lifestyle change* or *wellness*): my mom's wisdom about exercise and nutrition. The first was nonexistent. The word *aerobics* hadn't even been coined then, and weight loss was merely about food and eating. My mom's nutritional knowledge was basic and somewhat obvious—eliminate fried foods, sweets, and sugar. That was about it. I recall changing my diet and having many meals consisting of cheese on low-fat crackers. I switched to artificial sweeteners rather than sugar; and cut back on the beer, nuts, and fries. On my cheese-and-cracker diet, I actually lost the 30 pounds during the course of one summer.

Luckily, I knew the value of exercise, and in the summer of '74, I decided that in addition to eating lots of cheese, I also needed to increase my physical activity. So I began jogging on a regular basis. I got down to 180 pounds and maintained that weight, plus or minus about 5 pounds, for the next 20 years. Initially, my exercise was sporadic, but when I emigrated to America and became the clinical director of a wellness program, my jogging became a regular and enjoyable habit.

Along the way I've definitely changed my food preferences. At one time, I had a real sweet tooth, eating at least one candy bar every day. I still enjoy sweets, but now just a bite or two will suffice (if I indulge at all). I also had a very strong preference for table salt. It took me a long time to kick that habit, and just when I did, research suggested that salt may not be so bad after all!

For most of the 17 years that I've been in America, I've eaten healthfully and exercised sensibly. Still, when I changed my career several years ago, my weight started to rise just a little. I had left the wellness center and started public speaking, writing books, and developing my own practice full time. The change was as stressful as it was challenging, and I actually had less time for myself. Each time my weight crept up over 190, I'd be vigilant for a while and get it back down around 180 again, which, given my 6'1" height, is a reasonable weight. Within the last five years, however, my weight started to rise above 190.

There were times when, because of a variety of minor health issues, aches, and pains, my exercise would slip. At one time, there were questions about an abnormal EKG. Although my doctor assured me that there was nothing wrong, it made me apprehensive about pushing myself as much as I used to, and the exercise dipped further. I put it down to age and settled for a weight of 195 pounds.

Then, last year, I chartered a TOPS group in my hometown of Hilton Head, South Carolina. Obviously, I believe in the TOPS message and wanted to bring it to my own community. We started up just before Thanksgiving—a bold (some would even say foolhardy) maneuver. By January, few of us had lost much weight. When I got on the scale for the first time in the new year, I found myself in an unfamiliar territory at more than 200 pounds.

I have to admit to being shocked and annoyed at myself. Because of my frame and body type, very few people would consider me overweight even then, but I knew I was. What had happened? The fact was that I'd settled for a weight, as well as eating and exercise habits that I rationalized were acceptable for my age. I'd stopped paying attention and being vigilant. I liked to exercise, but it had become too easy to miss a few days—or even weeks—here and there.

I had no excuse this time. Unlike in college, I knew what to eat and how much was enough, and I knew what level of exercise was necessary to lose and maintain weight loss. Determined to stop rationalizing my excess weight and actually get on with doing what was necessary, I set my goal at 190 pounds, a weight I hadn't really maintained for a few years.

No, I didn't resort to cheese and low-fat crackers. I watched my portion sizes, replaced sodas and coffee with water, reduced the sweets, drastically cut back on junk food, and committed myself to exercise. I also discovered more about myself by doing something I hadn't really done before. . . .

Listen to Your Body

Somatic awareness refers to the process of listening to the body. Most of us aren't very good at this, only trying to do it when we suspect that there's something wrong with us. Yet there's much to be gained from learning how to accurately interpret physical sensations. Interesting research shows that many people report physical symptoms for which there are no obvious origins. Having been introduced to the concept of somatic aware-ness, I was interested in using it to help my weight-loss efforts. However, I was skeptical.

My first important lesson happened almost by chance. I decided that I'd fast for a whole day as an exercise in self-control. *What will happen,* I wondered, *if I don't eat for 24 hours?* This wasn't intended as a weight-management regimen, but an attempt to observe what would happen to my body if I didn't feed it.

Surprisingly, the fasting test didn't prove to be much of a challenge for my self-control. I started my fast in the evening, and I'd imagined that by the next afternoon I'd feel ravenous, possibly even light-headed, and that I'd certainly be lethargic and have a headache. To my amazement, I didn't even feel terribly hungry. Not only that, I was neither light-headed nor lethargic. On the contrary, I was productive, clear thinking, and energized. As the afternoon wore on, I was certainly aware that I hadn't eaten, but it was relatively easy to accept this hunger and move beyond it. To me, it was merely a physical sensation that could be managed.

As I considered the hunger puzzle, I had another important realiza-tion. I'd felt at least this hungry on days when I hit the snack machine in the middle of the afternoon. Occasionally, I'd grab something from the machine to boost my flagging energy. I discovered for myself what I knew intellectually, that typical snacks—a small candy bar, some nuts, snack mix, foods that were no more than a couple of hundred calories—actually make me feel *more* hungry. The reason for this is that blood-glucose levels can be quickly elevated with these foods, but when that level sinks, fatigue and lethargy result. That's why I never eat them (or much else for that matter) when driving long distances. My energy is higher and my focus is sharper when my blood-glucose level isn't bouncing all over the place.

Reaffirming that I could indeed survive hunger was also an important lesson. One of the rationalizations I'd used for eating, especially unhealthy foods, is that if I didn't eat, I would be hungry. So what? There's nothing wrong with being hungry. Being hungry is good for the soul. If I could face hunger and stay in control, then it would hold no fear for me. And if I wasn't afraid of hunger, then it would be a lot easier to manage appetite.

I also learned important lessons about exercise by listening to my body. As I've matured, different parts of my body have made it clear that they don't want to be ignored. My cartilage, tendons, and joints assert themselves by being painful, or simply making me aware of their presence.

In the past few years, I've used these aches and pains to justify limiting my level of exercise. When I really started to observe these minor ailments, however, I learned something very important: The aches and pains get worse when I *don't* exercise. If I stay with my regular routine and schedule, my body feels better than when I don't work out. The very evidence I used in the past as an excuse for being *inactive* is now motivation to be *active*. This is another example of the importance of evaluating old thinking habits. (Of course, I'm careful about staying within my routine and knowing my limitations. If I have more than minor pain, I will stop or take a day off, but this is rare.)

Matching physical sensations to moods and emotional states is also a valuable exercise, because physical sensations often reflect displaced emotions. Many people, for example, will focus on cardiac symptoms, such as palpitations, rather than consciously addressing the stress that's causing those symptoms. I've known several people who have rushed to the emergency room on the assumption that they were having a heart attack when they were actually having a panic attack. Tapping in to the body's wisdom is key to leading a healthy life.

Automatic Thinking

Much of what passes through our consciousness can be described as "automatic thinking habits." We develop views on certain topics, and they become unchallenged assumptions—we can have the same thoughts and perceptions for years and never bother to reevaluate them. Most people rarely check reality to see whether their thoughts are still valid or whether they've outgrown their usefulness. For example, I like to exercise first thing in the morning—it's a longtime habit. In fact, I began to assume that the morning was the only possible time to exercise. This notion had become second nature, but as soon as I made a concerted effort to evaluate my thoughts, I realized that there was absolutely no reason why I couldn't exercise in the afternoon or the evening. This might not be my preferred time, but to imagine that I could never exercise at a different hour was absurd.

Awareness of automatic thoughts and the ability to evaluate rather than automatically embrace what's going through your mind is an essential life skill. Just because a thought is passing through your head doesn't mean that you have to act upon it. For example, if a craving for chocolate suddenly strikes, you don't have to indulge it.

If you've enjoyed favorite foods for decades, then it's inevitable that you'll think about them longingly from time to time. The real issue is how you manage those thoughts once they pass through your mind. The various management strategies described in this book are all related to awareness of the consequences of acting out—feeling out of control, being depressed, letting yourself down, disappointing others, weight gain, and so on.

With healthier eating and a more reliable exercise schedule, I lost 20 pounds in six months. I moved my goal down from 190 to 185, a figure I previously imagined impossible. My weight now hovers between 180 and 185. I hadn't been in this kind of shape for at least ten years, probably longer. TOPS helped me a lot, and going to meetings made me accountable and kept me motivated. Half of the people in the group I belong to have dropped more than 20 pounds in the first half of this year.

For a while, my typical run was about four to five miles. I figured that much more than that might be damaging to my already sore knees, and the longer distances—the half marathon (13.1 miles) and marathon (26.2 miles)—were definitely beyond me.

A few weeks ago, however, on a glorious sunny day, I decided that rather than running for distance, I'd simply try to jog for 75 minutes. To my surprise, I made it fairly comfortably, matching the longest I'd ever run. I really didn't experience any ill effects, so the next week I decided to run for 90 minutes. Why not push the envelope? I'd be sensible—if it was too difficult, I'd simply stop and walk home.

As I ran past the hour mark, the thought occurred to me that if I continued to feel comfortable, I could go a little longer—maybe an hour and three quarters. When I hit 90 minutes, my legs were getting heavy but my breathing was fine, so I opted for an extra 15 minutes. Ten minutes later, the thought occurred to me that if I could run for two hours, I'd have effectively run a half marathon! Until that moment, such a distance hadn't seemed possible at all. So I ran for two hours and five minutes, which at my pace was close to the half-marathon distance of 13.1 miles. I'd achieved something I'd always thought was out of my reach, and I was ecstatic! I'd reached a goal that I'd considered all but impossible only 30 minutes earlier.

Extending my running in this way has changed how I think about my exercise. Now, five miles seems almost embarrassingly short. The knowledge that I can run for more than two hours has given me enormous confidence when exercising. In fact, two weeks ago I completed an official half marathon, along with 300 other runners from around the country. My old expectations have been replaced with newer ones that are more rewarding and challenging.

So my final message to you is *push the envelope*. Challenge yourself. Don't be confined by old habits, self-limiting thoughts, other people's neuroses, misguided intentions, or fear. Don't allow yourself to be controlled, sabotaged, threatened, persecuted, ridiculed, or humiliated by excess weight. Be courageous, determined, committed, focused, and resilient—like the contributors to this book. By acting in this way, you'll find the self-respect and self-care necessary for a fulfilling life. When you reach this point of self-acceptance, you'll find that peace, fulfillment, and meaning are not about food or even about weight—they're much bigger than that. They're about your relationships—with yourself, with other people, and with your God.

Good luck and go in peace.

"Love is the great miracle cure. Loving ourselves works miracles in our lives."

— Louise L. Hay, bestselling author

Take Off Pounds Sensibly— TOPS

❋

TOPS Club, Inc., is the oldest nonprofit, noncommercial weight-loss support group in the world, and it has more than 235,000 members across the globe. It was founded in 1948 by Esther Manz, a Milwaukee housewife who recognized the need for a support group to help people lose weight.

TOPS members lose weight sensibly through a combination of healthful dieting, exercise, realistic goal setting, and the support of other members. Since 1966, TOPS Club, Inc., has donated more than $5.4 million toward obesity research.

At the current time, membership is just $20 per year. This allows access to local meetings, which are held on a weekly basis, and subscription to *TOPS News,* a magazine about the organization and weight-loss support.

In addition to joining existing chapters, there are simple steps involved in starting your own group. The minimum number of people required to charter a new chapter is four. TOPS provides all the information needed to establish groups.

There are various ways to contact TOPS. Call 1-800-932-8677 for the location of the nearest chapter and a free brochure about Taking Off Pounds Sensibly, or visit the TOPS Website: **www.tops.org,** where you'll find the latest news about the organization and its members, current articles on weight loss and health, as well as information about local meetings. You can also write to: TOPS Club, Inc., 4575 Fifth St., Milwaukee, WI 53207-5800.

🌹 🌹 🌹

ABOUT THE AUTHOR

❧

A s the nationally acclaimed author of *Inspired to Lose, 7 Steps to Wellness, 10 Steps to a Great Relationship,* and *Power Talk: The Art of Effective Communication,* **Dr. Howard J. Rankin** is in demand wherever people want to learn how to take charge of their health and their lives.

Dr. Rankin's goal in both his writing and his highly celebrated seminars is to provide practical tools for overcoming life's obstacles. Through his research, academic background, and vast clinical experience, he teaches people to motivate, communicate, and develop resilience. His message effectively reaches large organizations as well as small groups.

Dr. Rankin is as comfortable doing stand-up comedy as he is delivering a serious keynote address. Using previous experience as a comedy writer, he's an entertaining and inspirational speaker. He has a natural ability to turn academic and research data into easily understood principles with real-life application (and he's the only person to have ever written a scientific paper in limerick form!). He has been described as "the best stand-up comedian in the serious subject of health," "a master communicator," and "the leading lifestyle-change expert."

Dr. Rankin's work has been featured on ABC's *20/20* as well as CNN and other television and radio shows. He's served as a consultant to the World Health Organization and the National Institute on Drug Abuse, and he's been featured in many newspapers and print media, including *The Wall Street Journal,* the *Los Angeles Times, The Baltimore Sun, The Dallas Morning News,* the *Cleveland Plain Dealer, Ladies' Home Journal, Prevention, Family Circle, Mademoiselle, Health, Woman's Day,* and *Weight Watchers* magazine, to name but a few.

Dr. Rankin can be reached at 843-842-7797, or by writing to P.O. Box 4797, Hilton Head Island, SC 29938, or at StepWisePress@aol.com. Website: **www.DrHowardRankin.com**.

HAY HOUSE TITLES OF RELATED INTEREST

Books

BodyChange™: The 21-Day Fitness Program for Changing Your Body . . .
and Changing Your Life! by Montel Williams and Wini Linguvic

Gut Feelings: From Fear and Despair to Health and Hope,
by Carnie Wilson, with Spotlight Health

I'm Still Hungry: Finding Myself Through Thick and Thin,
by Carnie Wilson, with Cindy Pearlman

Losing Your Pounds of Pain, by Doreen Virtue, Ph.D.

Love Your Body, by Louise L. Hay

Shape® Magazine's Shape Your Life: 4 Weeks to a Better Body—and a Better Life,
by Barbara Harris, editor-in-chief, *Shape* magazine, with Angela Hynes

Ultimate Pilates: Achieve the Perfect Body Shape, by Dreas Reyneke

Vegetarian Meals for People On-the-Go:
101 Quick & Easy Recipes, by Vimala Rodgers

The Yo-Yo Diet Syndrome: How to Heal and Stabilize Your
Appetite and Weight, by Doreen Virtue, Ph.D.

Card Decks

I Can Do It® Cards, by Louise L. Hay

Power Thought Cards, by Louise L. Hay

Self-Care Cards, by Cheryl Richardson

Tips for Daily Living Cards, by Iyanla Vanzant

All of the above are available at your local
bookstore, or may be ordered by visiting:
Hay House USA: **www.hayhouse.com**
Hay House Australia: **www.hayhouse.com.au**
Hay House UK: **www.hayhouse.co.uk**
Hay House South Africa: **orders@psdprom.co.za**

❧ ❧ ❧

We hope you enjoyed this Hay House book.
If you would like to receive a free catalog featuring
additional Hay House books and products, or if you would
like information about the Hay Foundation, please contact:

Hay House, Inc.
P.O. Box 5100
Carlsbad, CA 92018-5100

(760) 431-7695 or (800) 654-5126
(760) 431-6948 (fax) or (800) 650-5115 (fax)
www.hayhouse.com

❧ ❧ ❧

Published and distributed in Australia by:
Hay House Australia Pty. Ltd. • 18/36 Ralph St. • Alexandria NSW 2015
Phone: 612-9669-4299 • *Fax:* 612-9669-4144 • www.hayhouse.com.au

Published and distributed in the United Kingdom by:
Hay House UK, Ltd. • Unit 62, Canalot Studios
222 Kensal Rd., London W10 5BN • *Phone:* 44-20-8962-1230
Fax: 44-20-8962-1239 • www.hayhouse.co.uk

Published and distributed in the Republic of South Africa by:
Hay House SA (Pty), Ltd., P.O. Box 990, Witkoppen 2068
Phone/Fax: 2711-7012233 • orders@psdprom.co.za

Distributed in Canada by: Raincoast
9050 Shaughnessy St., Vancouver, B.C. V6P 6E5
Phone: (604) 323-7100 • *Fax:* (604) 323-2600

❧ ❧ ❧

Sign up via the Hay House USA Website to receive the Hay House online
newsletter and stay informed about what's going on with your favorite authors.
You'll receive bimonthly announcements about: Discounts and Offers, Special
Events, Product Highlights, Free Excerpts, Giveaways, and more!
www.hayhouse.com

❧ ❧ ❧